FIRST AID

FOR THE®
MATCH

Fourth Edition

TAO LE, MD, MHS

Assistant Clinical Professor of Medicine and Pediatrics
Division of Allergy and Clinical Immunology
University of Louisville

VIKAS BHUSHAN, MD

Diagnostic Radiologist

APRIL TROY, MPH

Johns Hopkins University School of Medicine
Class of 2007

McGraw-Hill
MEDICAL PUBLISHING DIVISION

New York / Chicago / San Francisco / Lisbon / London /
Milan / New Delhi / San Juan / Seoul / Singapore / Sydr

First Aid for the® Match, Fourth Edition

1 2 3 4 5 6 7 8 9 0 QPD/QPD 0 9 8 7 6

ISBN-13: 978-0-07-147291-3
ISBN-10: 0-07-147291-6
ISSN: 1090-364X

This book was set in Electra LH by Rainbow Graphics.
The editor was Catherine A. Johnson.
The production supervisor was Phil Galea.
Production management was provided by Rainbow Graphics.
Quebecor Dubuque was printer and binder.

This book is printed on acid-free paper.

DEDICATION

To the contributors of this and past editions, who took time to share their experience, advice, and humor for the benefit of future physicians.

and

To our families, friends, and loved ones, who supported us in the task of assembling this guide.

CONTENTS

CHAPTER 6   GETTING RESIDENCY INFORMATION AND APPLICATIONS   111

CHAPTER 7   THE APPLICATION   129

CHAPTER 8   THE CURRICULUM VITAE   147

CHAPTER 9   THE PERSONAL STATEMENT   161

AUTHORS

Rachel Brennan, MD
Resident in Pediatrics
Johns Hopkins University

Alissa Brown, MD
Resident in Pediatrics
Children's Hospital of Pittsburgh

Jessica M. Ghaferi, MD
Resident in Dermatology
Henry Ford Medical Center

Chad A. Glazer, MD
Resident in Otolaryngology Head and Neck Surgery
Johns Hopkins University

Rajesh Jari, MD, MSc
Resident in Physical Medicine and Rehabilitation
Johns Hopkins University

Katherine Stabenow, MD
Resident in Pediatrics
Johns Hopkins University

PREFACE

With the fourth edition of *First Aid for the® Match*, we continue our commitment to providing students and international medical graduates (IMGs) with the most useful and up-to-date information to help guide them through the residency application and interview process and obtain a residency position in the specialty of their choice. The fourth edition represents a thorough revision and includes:

- The latest insider advice from students who have successfully made it through the 2006 National Residency Matching Program (NRMP) Match
- Up-to-date information and statistics from the NRMP Match, including the latest trends in each of the specialty fields
- A revised and expanded chapter on advice for IMGs
- Updated specialty coverage, including specialty trends in education, research, and clinical practice
- An expanded guide to the Electronic Residency Application Service (ERAS)
- Top residency application mistakes and how to avoid them
- A revised, in-depth travel advice section, with detailed information on discount airfares and hotel lodging, as well as descriptions of many unique online travel and lodging sites
- An extensive compilation of commonly asked interview questions, broken down by specialty

The fourth edition would not have been possible without the help of dedicated students and faculty members, who contributed their feedback and suggestions. We invite both students and faculty to share their thoughts and ideas to help us continue to improve *First Aid for the® Match* in the future. (See How to Contribute, p. xvii.)

Louisville	Tao Le
Los Angeles	Vikas Bhushan
Baltimore	April Troy

ACKNOWLEDGMENTS

This has been a collaborative project from the start. We gratefully acknowledge the thoughtful comments and advice of the residents, international medical graduates, and faculty who have supported the authors in the development of *First Aid for the® Match*.

For support and encouragement throughout the process, we are grateful to Thao Pham and Jonathan Kirsch. We owe a special thanks to Selina Bush and Louise Peterson for their administrative assistance during this revision. Thanks to our publisher, McGraw-Hill, for the valuable assistance of their staff. For enthusiasm, support, and commitment to this challenging project, thanks to our editor, Catherine Johnson. For outstanding editorial work, we thank Susan Early. A special thanks to Rainbow Graphics for remarkable production work.

Louisville	Tao Le
Los Angeles	Vikas Bhushan
Baltimore	April Troy

HOW TO CONTRIBUTE

First Aid for the® Match incorporates many contributions and changes from students and faculty. We invite you to participate in this process. In addition, we offer **paid internships** in medical education (please see below). Please send us:

- Strategies for applying and interviewing in your specialty
- Your personal statement and CV (feel free to edit or mask for privacy)
- Anecdotes of your application and interviewing experiences
- Your medical school's guide to the Match
- Corrections and clarifications

Personalized contributions (i.e., anecdotes and personal statements), if used, will be altered to protect the identity of the contributor. For entries incorporated into the next edition, you will receive an Amazon.com gift certificate and personal acknowledgment in the next edition. Significant contributions will be compensated at the discretion of the authors.

The preferred way to submit suggestions and corrections is via electronic mail, addressed to:

firstaidteam@yahoo.com

Otherwise, you can send entries, neatly written or typed or on disk (Microsoft Word), to:

First Aid Team
914 North Dixie Avenue, Suite 100
Elizabethtown, KY 42701
Attention: Match Contributions

All entries become property of the authors and are subject to editing and reviewing. Please verify all data and spellings carefully. In the event that similar or duplicate entries are received, only the first entry received will be used. Please follow the style, punctuation, and format of this edition if possible.

INTERNSHIP OPPORTUNITIES

The author is pleased to offer part-time and full-time paid internships in medical education and publishing to motivated medical students and physicians. Internships may range from two to three months (e.g., a summer) up to a full year. Participants will have an opportunity to author, edit, and earn academic credit on a wide variety of projects, including the popular *First Aid* series. Writing/editing experience, familiarity with Microsoft Word, and Internet access are desired. For more information, e-mail a résumé or a short description of your experience along with a cover letter to **firstaidteam@yahoo.com**.

CHAPTER 1

The Match

Preparing for the Match is a time to celebrate! Graduation is in sight, and opportunities abound. With this wide variety of opportunities, however, comes responsibility. Choosing a residency position is likely to be more complicated than choosing a university or medical school. Postgraduate education may be seen by many as more of an uncharted sea. More than 31,000 students will compete in the Match, and there will be over 25,000 rank-order lists (ROLs). You will therefore need to plan your senior year carefully and be prepared to make decisions on a strict timetable. Once you have chosen your specialty, you must obtain program information and applications. In addition, senior electives must be scheduled to coincide with the application and interview process, and a personal statement and curriculum vitae (CV) must be written in conjunction with adviser meetings. A well-thought-out plan of action for the senior year will maximize your likelihood of success. Fortunately, faculty, colleagues, and advisers have seen the process evolve year after year, sharing in students' successes and remembering their mistakes. Presented below are the suggestions, advice, and experience of students, residents, and deans. We look forward to helping you chart this great sea of opportunity called the Match.

Students' two biggest fears are (1) not matching at any program; and (2) ending up in a program that is not right for them. Approximately 6.3% of U.S. students, 27.1% of Canadian participants, and 44.4% of non-U.S. foreign graduates in the National Resident Matching Program (NRMP) went without a matched position on the big day in 2005. Conversely, almost 8% of available NRMP positions remained unfilled.

A number of common mistakes that medical students make year after year result in an unmatched or a poor-choice position. This guide will help students avoid mistakes such as:

- **Not understanding the details of the Match for a particular specialty.** For example, for some specialties, a preliminary year must be secured along with the specialty program. Some programs have their own match process as well as an earlier timetable for each step of the senior-year plan.
- **Starting the application process too late.** One step follows another, and a late start can result in more interviews in the winter months than can actually be accomplished.
- **Applying to or ranking too few programs to ensure a match.** By the time a student realizes that he or she has been invited to only a few interviews, it may be too late to add program applications.
- **Not seeking adequate counseling and advice.** No student is an island in the match process. Independent thinking and individualism may be admired in the medical profession, but the residency Match requires input from a variety of sources, including publications, advisers, colleagues, and word of mouth.
- **Inadequate preparation and understanding of the role of interviews, personal statements, and CVs.** Learn about these instruments through the eyes of those who use them to rank students.
- **Unclear goals and expectations.** Most students have the necessary credentials for acceptance into excellent programs. However, students must work to find the right programs, focus on the programs of choice, and define what they are really looking for in a residency program.

- **Becoming overly confident during the application process.** Many programs will be very positive about the applicant. Some candidates, however, will misinterpret compliments about their record as a guarantee of a match.
- A small number of students who do not match may miss out on many opportunities that are briefly available during "Scramble Day." These students need intense assistance and counseling at a strategic time in the process.

WHAT IS THE MATCH?

Although there are actually several matches, most people know the NRMP as the Match. While the NRMP offers positions in a wide range of specialties, some specialties use their own match, such as neurology, neurosurgery, ophthalmology, and urology (see Table 1-1). With more than 90% of all graduating U.S. and Canadian medical students participating, along with a surprisingly high number of international medical graduates (IMGs), the NRMP is the largest match by far (see Figure 1-1).

The basic modus operandi of the Match is as follows: After the interview season, residency training programs submit a list of applicants in the order in which they would offer acceptances, and students enter lists of programs in the order in which they would accept offers. Both students and programs then submit their rankings to the NRMP. Subsequently, in a matter of minutes, a computer program matches each student to the highest program on his or her

TABLE 1-1. Specialties with Their Own Matches

SPECIALTY	MATCHING PROGRAM	MONTH OF MATCH DAY	WEB SITE
Neurosurgery	Neurological Surgery Matching Program P.O. Box 45161 San Francisco, CA 94145-0161 (415) 447-0350 Fax: (415) 561-8535	January of senior year	http://www.sfmatch.org help@SFmatch.org
Ophthalmology	Ophthalmology Matching Program P.O. Box 45161 San Francisco, CA 94145-0161 (415) 447-0350 Fax: (415) 561-8535	January of senior year	http://www.sfmatch.org help@SFmatch.org
Urology	AUA Residency Matching Program 1000 Corporate Boulevard Linthicum, MD 21090 (866) 746-4282, ext. 3913 Fax: (410) 689-3939	January of senior year	http://www.auanet.org resmatch@auanet.org

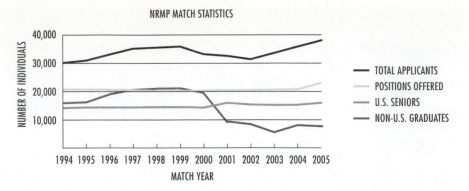

NRMP MATCH STATISTICS

— TOTAL APPLICANTS
— POSITIONS OFFERED
— U.S. SENIORS
— NON-U.S. GRADUATES

FIGURE 1-1. Applicants in the NRMP Match

FIGURE 1-2. Flowchart of the NRMP Match, based on 2005 NRMP Match data.

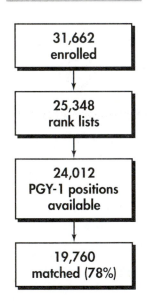

31,662
enrolled

25,348
rank lists

24,012
PGY-1 positions
available

19,760
matched (78%)

The Match brought order to a

chaotic process.

list that offered a position. The Match usually occurs in late February, and its results are announced simultaneously across the country on "Match Day" in mid-March. In 2005, 31,662 applicants enrolled in the Match, and of the 25,348 applicants who submitted ROLs, 19,760 received offers (see Figure 1-2). This translates into an overall match rate of 78% into a PGY-1 residency program.

If you are a U.S. medical student, you will automatically receive information about the NRMP Match through your school during the spring of your third year. However, the NRMP can be contacted directly for more information at:

National Resident Matching Program
2450 N Street, N.W.
Washington, D.C. 20037-1127
(202) 828-0676 for U.S. seniors
(202) 828-0566 for independent applicants
www.nrmp.org

WHY IS THERE A MATCH?

The Match exists in the form that we know it today to provide a semblance of order to an otherwise seemingly chaotic process of matching thousands of medical graduates with residency programs across the spectrum of specialties. Before a formal matching process was instituted in 1952 both applicants and programs were not given a fair opportunity to explore all of their options. Less competitive programs tried to get a head start by asking applicants to commit to their programs early in the fourth and sometimes even third year of medical school. Students were forced to gamble—i.e., to decide whether to accept an early offer from a less competitive program, thereby forfeiting a later shot at better programs, or to pass up the early offer and risk not being accepted in a better program that offered positions later after sifting through a larger pool of applicants. Residency directors faced a similar dilemma in the fact that if they filled their positions too quickly, they would not be able to offer spots to more attractive applicants. The 1952 Match was a huge success; for the first time, applicants and programs were able to rank each other on the basis of desirability without being forced to make hasty decisions. The algorithm used to match applicants with programs has remained largely unchanged over the years (see Chapter 12).

Although the NRMP is the largest matching program available to U.S. medical students and IMGs, there are other matches as well, including some that operate independently of the NRMP.

Specialties with Their Own Matches

Some specialties have their own match processes with different match days. These specialties include neurosurgery, ophthalmology, and urology. Since many of these specialties require training in medicine, pediatrics, or surgery, most applicants also match through the NRMP for one or two years of transitional training before starting their specialty work. Many students aiming for these specialties also apply for another specialty in the NRMP Match as a backup (e.g., general surgery as a backup for neurosurgery). Please refer to Chapter 4 for more specific matching information regarding your target specialty.

NRMP Couples Match

In the couples Match, the NRMP allows any two people to be matched with residency programs in the same geographic area if they so desire. Any two people can apply as a couple. Partners apply and interview separately at programs in the same geographic region. They then submit an ROL of pairs of programs in the order in which they would accept offers. Because couples are often limited by geographic constraints, they frequently submit more applications to maximize the likelihood of achieving a successful match. To help matters, the ROL gives a couple the option of seeking matches in separate locations or allowing one partner to go unmatched in the event that a couples match is not possible.

Any two people can apply as a couple.

Some residency directors and deans believe that many couples do better together in the Match than they would if they applied and matched separately. Couples tend to be viewed as more stable and less likely to leave residency programs. Given the hassles involved in moving again after residency, especially with kids, couples are also regarded as more likely to contribute to the faculty pool of the institution in which they trained. Nevertheless, the results of the couples match can be unpredictable, especially when both people are applying to competitive programs. In addition, couples tend to seek reassurance from their interviewers that everything will turn out well and may thus be particularly prone to misinterpret encouragement as a guarantee about the match result. For more information about the couples match, consult the section on "Special Cases" in your NRMP Handbook for Students or consult the NRMP Web site (www.nrmp.org).

Shared-Schedule Match

A few programs in the Match offer shared-residency positions. Shared-schedule positions in the NRMP Match allow two people to share the duties and responsibilities of one residency position. An applicant enrolls individually in the NRMP Match and then pairs up with a partner by completing a Shared Residency Pair Form, due in the fall preceding Match Day. The pair shares one NRMP applicant code, applies and interviews together, and submits a single ROL. Although each person will spend less than full time working (e.g., alternate months on rotation), both will spend more time in residency and will eventually do as much work as, if not more work than, a full-time resident. Many applicants seek shared-schedule positions because of family responsibilities or research, among other reasons. When a pair is matched to a position, both are bound to accept it. With the enforcement of 80-hour workweeks, such paired programs may become even less common. Consult "Special Cases" in your NRMP Handbook for Students for more information or consult the NRMP Web site (www.nrmp.org).

Canadian Match

The Canadian Resident Matching Service (CaRMS) was founded in 1970. Like its U.S. counterpart, the CaRMS Match is an orderly approach toward matching applicants to their top choices and residency programs to their preferred applicants. In fact, the CaRMS uses the same matching algorithm as the NRMP, although its Match Day is in mid-February. Approximately 1400 Canadian students apply for roughly 1500 slots annually offered through the Canadian Match. The CaRMS is an eight-month process that includes an application cycle, an interview period, a ranking period, and match result announcements. The CaRMS is open to U.S. seniors, although few apply. In September, applicants are sent a unique token by e-mail to initiate their application by the Applicant Webstation. Most graduating Canadian medical students participate in the First Iteration Match. In addition, 700 "independent" applicants compete for approximately 200 positions available in the Second Iteration Match. Independent applicants include former graduates of Canadian medical schools, U.S. students, and graduates of international medical schools. For more information, contact:

Canadian Resident Matching Service
2283 St. Laurent Boulevard, Suite 110
Ottawa, Ontario, Canada K1G 3H7
(613) 237-0075
Fax: (613) 563-2860
www.carms.ca/jsp/main.jsp
help@carms.ca

Osteopathic Match

The AOA Intern/Resident Registration Program, the osteopathic version of the Match, is run by the National Matching Services Inc. (NMS). All osteopathic graduates are required to take a one-year osteopathic rotating internship approved by the American Osteopathic Association (AOA) before entering an osteopathic residency. Applicants interview in late summer and fall, submit an ROL by late January, and await results on the osteopathic Match Day in mid-February.

Approximately 2200 osteopathic internships and 1100 residency positions are offered through the osteopathic match every year. Osteopathic residency directors have recently had more difficulty filling their positions, as osteopathic graduates have gained wider acceptance in allopathic residency programs, and the AOA has relaxed its restrictions on osteopathic graduates pursuing allopathic training through the NRMP Match. The AOA opportunities database of internship and residency positions is available on the AOA's Web site at www.do-online.org (select the option for students and residents). For more information, contact:

American Osteopathic Association
Department of Education
142 East Ontario Street
Chicago, IL 60611
(800) 621-1773, ext. 7426
Fax: (312) 202-8200
www.do-online.osteotech.org
info@osteotech.org

National Matching Services
Box 1208
Lewiston, NY 14092-8208
(716) 282-4013
Fax: (716) 282-0611

National Matching Services
20 Holly Street, Suite 301
Toronto, Ontario, Canada M453B1
(416) 977-3431
Fax: (416) 977-5020

Armed Forces Match

Army, Navy, and Air Force residencies conduct their own matching process early in the senior year, several months before the NRMP Match takes place. Applicants usually have military service obligations (e.g., graduates of the Uniformed Services University of the Health Sciences School of Medicine and participants in the Health Professions Scholarship Program). After senior-year applicants have been interviewed, the military programs convene in late November and early December each year to match programs and applicants in a week-long affair known as "Selection Boards." Many students apply to both matches using the NRMP as a fallback, particularly when a competitive military program is sought. Students who do not match successfully in a military program can usually begin interviewing late as long as initial applications have been completed. All medical graduates of the Uniformed Services University are preferentially placed through an Armed Forces match. If you match with a military residency program, you are obliged to withdraw from the NRMP Match or from any other civilian match.

For more information on the Army military match, contact the regional Army Medical Department (AMEDD) counselor. For more information on the Air Force military match, contact:

Headquarters AFPC/DPAME
550 C Street West, Suite 27
Randolph Air Force Base, TX 78150-4729
(800) 531-5800
DSN 487-6331

For more information on the Navy military match, contact:

Bureau of Medicine and Surgery
2300 E Street, N.W.
Washington, D.C. 20372-5300
(202) 653-1318

TABLE 1-2. Success of U.S. Seniors in the NRMP Match

Choice Obtained	Percent of U.S. Seniors (2000)	Percent of U.S. Seniors (2001)	Percent of U.S. Seniors (2002)	Percent of U.S. Seniors (2003)	Percent of U.S. Seniors (2004)	Percent of U.S. Seniors (2005)
First	62.4	61.0	61.0	62.4	61.9	62.5
Second	15.3	15.6	15.5	15.7	15.6	15.0
Third	8.7	8.7	9.4	8.4	8.6	8.7
Fourth	4.8	5.1	5.0	5.2	4.8	4.7
> Fourth	8.8	9.6	9.1	8.3	9.0	9.1

WHAT ARE MY CHANCES OF SUCCESS IN THE MATCH?

Table 1-3. 2005 NRMP Match Rate

Applicant Type	PGY-1 Match Rate (%)
U.S. seniors	93.7
Canadian students	72.9
U.S. graduates	44.3
Osteopaths	68.6
U.S. citizen foreign graduates	54.7
Non-U.S. foreign graduates	55.6

In general, U.S. seniors do well in the NRMP Match. Roughly 85% of U.S. seniors obtain one of their first three choices each year (see Table 1-2). The U.S. senior nonmatch rate has held steady at 6–7% for the past ten years and was 6.3% in 2005. In contrast, other applicants fare rather poorly (see Table 1-3). In the 2005 Match, only 44.3% of U.S. graduates (as opposed to U.S. seniors) and 55.6% of IMGs in the NRMP were successfully matched. IMGs, whether U.S. citizens or not, generally fare the worst.

HOW DO I REGISTER FOR THE NRMP MATCH?

U.S. Seniors

A U.S. senior is defined as one who has attended a Liaison Committee on Medical Education (LCME)-accredited school and is on schedule for graduation the year of the Match. Registration occurs online through the NRMP Web site, www.nrmp.org/res_match. The system uses the Association of American Medical Colleges (AAMC) ID along with a password that can be assigned during registration. Students are asked to review the terms of the Match agreement and the policies of the NRMP.

Payment of the registration fee also occurs online through use of a credit card number. As stated by the NRMP, registration entitles the user to access to the NRMP site, the processing of up to 15 program ranks and 15 ranks on the supplemental ROLs (SROLs), and access to a restricted Web site that lists unfilled positions. An additional $30 is assessed for each program added to your ROL after you have selected 15 programs.

Independent Applicants

The category of "independent applicant" includes several groups: previous graduates of a U.S. medical school, Canadian students/graduates, osteopathic students/graduates, students of a fifth-pathway program, and IMGs. Registration is online and follows the same method as that for U.S. seniors. You will be asked to select the correct category of application. The NRMP will collect information to verify eligibility, including United States Medical Licensing Examination/Educational Commission for Foreign Medical Graduates (USMLE/ECFMG) identification number in the case of IMGs.

The NRMP requires that foreign graduates pass all exams necessary for ECFMG certification, including the Clinical Skills Assessment. Independent applicant names should be exactly the same as those used by the Electronic Residency Application Service (ERAS) and the ECFMG. Payment is also on-line, and registration entitles independent applicants to the same benefits as U.S. seniors.

WHAT ABOUT THE OTHER MATCHES?

If you are a U.S. medical student, information pamphlets and registration materials for specialties outside the NRMP Match should be available at your dean's office. Otherwise, you can contact the specialty match programs directly for information and registration forms (see Table 1-1). To register for the armed forces Match, contact your military branch's medical personnel counselor or your local armed forces recruitment officer. **Don't forget to register for the NRMP Match regardless of what other matches you enroll in.** Nothing prevents you from enrolling in multiple matches; you just can't accept more than one appointment. Many non-NRMP matches require a preliminary transitional year obtained through the NRMP Match. In addition, many of these matches are highly competitive, and the NRMP Match is a nice backup. It's better to register, match in advance, and lose the $65 fee than to find yourself unable to participate in the Match at all.

Always enroll in the NRMP Match as a backup regardless of what other matches interest you.

NRMP PUBLICATIONS

The NRMP offers a wealth of valuable publications that few students know about and fewer still take the time to read. A handbook and the NRMP Directory are provided online in the Register/Log-in area to registered participants. The rest can be ordered from the NRMP by calling (202) 828-0416 or by filling out the NRMP publications order form found in the back of the NRMP Directory and mailing it to:

Attention: Membership and Publication Orders
National Resident Matching Program
2450 N Street, N.W.
Washington, D.C. 20037-1127

You can also order NRMP publications through the NRMP Web site at www.nrmp.org. Each NRMP publication is listed below.

NRMP Handbook for Students

The NRMP Handbook for Students is available free of charge through U.S. medical schools and is aimed at U.S. seniors and sponsored graduates. Read it from cover to cover, as it thoroughly describes the NRMP and its role in the residency application process. You will be able to decipher the NRMP philosophy despite the stilted prose. The handbook includes current details for registering for the Match and describes the couples match and shared-residency positions. It also supplies concise explanations for ROLs and SROLs. However, some of the juiciest information in the handbook can be found in its appendices, which include selected statistics from the previous

Match, NRMP policy statements, and an explanation of the Match algorithm. Finally, the handbook's back cover lists key dates applicable to the Match process.

NRMP Handbook for Independent Applicants

Like the NRMP Handbook for Students, this free publication from the NRMP is a must-read for independent applicants. You can get a copy by calling the NRMP at (202) 828-0566. The version for independent applicants covers the same topics as the general student handbook. In addition, the Handbook for Independent Applicants contains guidelines for the verification of credentials for Match eligibility, an NRMP publications order form, and Match dates for specialties covered in the NRMP's Specialties Matching Services.

NRMP Directory/Hospitals and Programs Participating in the Matching Program

The NRMP Directory is a catalog of residency programs participating in the Match. Part I of the directory organizes the programs by hospital. Use this section to see what other specialty training programs are offered at the hospitals you're interested in. For example, since the presence of an internal medicine program typically means a lower caliber of training for family practice residents, family practice applicants may want to find hospitals without internal medicine programs. Part II lists programs by specialty type and is much more useful. You should receive the edition for the previous Match at no cost upon registration. You will also receive a revised edition for your Match year late in the fall.

NRMP Program Results/Listing of Filled and Unfilled Programs for the Match

If you want to find out which programs in your specialty were not filled last year, this is the book to get. It's like going through someone's dirty laundry. The NRMP Program Results book is distributed on Unmatch Day to unmatched applicants, who must then enter the Scramble. Part II lists programs that did not fill all their spots. This can be a real eye-opener and can also give you a better feel for regional trends in competitiveness. If you are a marginal candidate applying in a competitive specialty, you may want to consider applying to several of the programs that went unfilled last year. But be forewarned—these programs probably went unfilled for good reason. Although this publication is supposedly free of charge only to applicants who failed to find placements in the previous Match, you can check your school's student affairs office for a copy.

Have a look at the NRMP data. The results may suprise you.

NRMP Data

This must-have publication contains exhaustive data on the previous year's Match. It tracks Match trends over several years and puts you and your target specialty into perspective. Many of the tables are informative, but you'll want to check out a few choice ones (see Table 1-4). Most students erroneously believe that Match data are confidential. In point of fact, they aren't if you can

TABLE 1-4. Must-See Tables/Charts in the NRMP Data Book

TABLES/CHARTS	WHAT TO LOOK FOR
Applicants in the matching program	Detailed Match statistics, grouped by applicant category. Compares U.S. seniors to foreign graduates.
PGY-1 positions, active applicants, and match rates	Presents similar information as previous table, but in the context of the number of PGY-1 positions available.
Positions offered and % filled by U.S. seniors and total applicants	Breaks down Match fill rates over the previous five years by specialty. Allows you to spot trends in each specialty.
Programs, positions, ranked and filled	The rank/position value is the average number of times each position offered by that specialty was ranked. A rank/position value roughly corresponds to the degree of competitiveness—the higher the number, the tougher it is to get the spot.
U.S. seniors unmatched	Highlights the specialties in which students have had the most difficulty matching.

come up with $7 plus shipping or if you consult the copy in your school's student affairs office. Unfortunately, many student affairs offices operate on the belief that these data are confidential or that students don't really need such details.

Universal Application for Residency and Program Designation Card

You get one or two Universal Applications free when you sign up for the Match. There should be no need to purchase additional copies. Because you send a photocopy of the Universal Application to the few programs that accept it, simply photocopy your application if you need more copies (i.e., as a worksheet). For detailed advice on completing the Universal Application, see Chapter 7. Programs that are ERAS or are under the SF Match do not use the Universal Application.

Program Designation and Acknowledgment Card

This self-addressed card to acknowledge receipt of your application is a bit lame, as it has no space for the program secretary to acknowledge receipt of other materials, such as letters of recommendation and medical school transcripts. You can easily design a more useful acknowledgment card yourself (see application status postcard, p. 145). One free card comes with your Universal Application.

References

National Resident Matching Program. *Advanced Copy of Results and Data, 2005 Match.* Washington, D.C., 2005.

National Resident Matching Program. *Handbook for U.S. Medical Students, 2005 Match.* Washington, D.C., 2005.

National Resident Matching Program. *NRMP Data: 2005.* Washington, D.C., 2005.

National Resident Matching Program Web site. http://www.nrmp.org/res_match/data_tables.html.

CHAPTER 2

Setting Up the Fourth Year

Despite what you have heard from friends and colleagues, the fourth year of medical school is full of events and deadlines for graduation, application, and the Match. It is also a time to expand your experiences both inside and outside the hospital or clinic. Although these dual purposes seem contradictory, they can both be achieved with some advance planning. In arranging the fourth year, however, you need to arm yourself with tools with which to navigate the residency application process from start to finish. For a maximally fulfilling and successful fourth year, you must also take advantage of the resources that surround you at your medical school and beyond. The first step is to find an adviser.

HOW DO I PICK AN ADVISER?

During your first three years of medical school, you may have identified or been assigned an academic adviser who shepherded you through a variety of situations, from surviving gross anatomy to helping you choose a medical specialty. If your adviser is an internist and you want to go into internal medicine, you may already be in great shape. However, if you choose a field that differs from that of your adviser or if your adviser does not closely monitor your application and matching process, you will need someone else to provide you with additional advice.

An adviser should be both counselor and advocate.

In selecting an adviser, you should seek someone who is savvy about a wide variety of factors regarding your career choice and the Match (see Figure 2-1). Your adviser should be able to keep you informed of both academic and economic trends as well as training and job opportunities in your chosen field. He or she should be familiar with the strong and weak points of your candidacy and should know you well enough to offer personal, honest advice. You should also seek an adviser who is familiar with the programs in which you are interested. For example, an adviser who trained on the East Coast may not be familiar with West Coast programs. Similarly, if you are interested in academic medicine, you should not choose an adviser who is primarily involved in private practice (or vice versa). Your adviser should be able to answer a range of questions about the application process, from matters of fact (When are the deadlines?) to advice (Whom should I ask for recommendations?). Some students even advocate a dual-adviser system: one adviser to assist you with the "nuts and bolts" of the process and another more senior, well-known faculty member whose connections and telephone lobbying might open more doors for you.

FIGURE 2-1. Checklist for the career adviser.

☐ Discuss current academic and economic trends in the field
☐ Point out research opportunities
☐ Provide overall view of the application process
☐ Offer honest assessment of your competitive standing
☐ Highlight programs most appropriate for you
☐ Review and critique your application (e.g., personal statement, CV)
☐ Conduct a mock interview
☐ Review your rank-order list
☐ Make key "political" phone calls if necessary
☐ Be available on Unmatch Day

How do you find such an adviser? Start by asking students in the class ahead of you about outstanding faculty members in your discipline. Your current medical school adviser may also have some suggestions. The dean of students can often guide you to the appropriate advisers. Ask the department chair or the residency director at your school whom they would recommend. The best advisers are junior or senior faculty members who are involved in residency selection and who have advised applicants in previous years. In the process of identifying your ideal adviser, however, you should be aware of the following potential pitfalls:

- **Adviser overload:** A person who counsels so many students that you're left with little attention (this can also be a problem with faculty who write many recommendation letters each year).
- **Adviser oversight:** A person who tends to misjudge a student's competitiveness or the competitiveness of the field.
- **Adviser nostalgia:** A faculty member who remembers what it was like in your field many years ago but who no longer has an accurate perception of the Match.
- **Adviser bias:** One who gives all students the same "pet" list of programs to apply to regardless of their personal career goals, their geographic constraints, or the strength of their candidacy.

Some students also make the mistake of sticking with a mentor with whom they worked on a research project during the first two years of medical school. Often, this choice is made out of fear that your former mentor will be insulted if he or she is excluded from your residency plans. Such faculty members, however, may or may not be the best advisers for you, especially if they are not actively involved in the residency application process at your school. So bear in mind that a mentor does not always make the best adviser, just as race car drivers don't always make the best driving instructors.

WHEN SHOULD I SCHEDULE MY ACTING INTERNSHIPS?

On the inside front cover is a checklist/time line for organizing Match activities during your fourth year in medical school. Conventional wisdom says that you should do at least one acting internship (or AI, aka subinternship, externship, junior internship, or senior clerkship) in your target specialty early in your fourth year (or late in your third year at some schools). Your evaluation during this rotation is one of the most influential factors the selection committee will consider. In addition, a strong letter of recommendation from an attending physician on this rotation is usually critical to a competitive application. Some programs will expect at least one letter of recommendation from an AI (if you did one) as part of your application. Verify with the dean's office the last rotation block that will show up in your dean's letter and on your transcript (usually September).

An additional factor to consider is that several specialties—most notably surgical subspecialties such as neurosurgery and orthopedics—effectively require an "in-house" rotation if a student is to be considered at that program. See Chapter 4 for the trends in each specialty, and also refer to the discussion on audition rotations below.

Given the importance of this rotation, many students like to do a "warm-up" rotation before going all out on the AI. Students interested in internal medicine, for example, often rotate on cardiology, infectious disease, or emergency medicine before beginning an internal medicine AI. This warm-up rotation allows you to acquire the experience, knowledge, and skills (both political and manual) that are necessary for success on your AI. The rotation also ensures that you will enter the AI refreshed and enthusiastic. Don't relax *too* much, however, as strong grades or evaluations within electives of your target specialty are also highly regarded by selection committees. Students interested in surgical specialties (e.g., orthopedics, neurosurgery) often elect to do a general surgery AI before beginning an AI in their specific interest in order to hone their floor management and operating room skills.

If you choose to do a second AI, either by requirement or by desire, note that there are good reasons for doing them early as well as for postponing them (see Table 2-1).

An AI is a great way to impress faculty and residency directors, but what if you feel that you don't need one? If you feel you are a stellar applicant and are applying in a less competitive field, it may not be worth the cost and hassle to move across the country for three weeks just to get a couple of nice paragraphs added to your already strong dean's letter. Consider doing your AI at home, but first talk with your adviser before you cement any plans.

WHEN SHOULD I SCHEDULE TIME FOR INTERVIEWS?

For the majority of students, interview dates run from November to early February. Students participating in "early matches" (e.g., neurosurgery, urology, ophthalmology) should leave time for interviews in November and early December. Most students take a month off for interviews starting right before or after Christmas break. Note, however, that unless you are considering a smaller number of programs in a limited geographic area, a two-week Christmas break is usually not enough. That said, you should keep in mind that with the exception of your AI, most of your fourth year will consist of elective time. These rotations expect a degree of absenteeism from fourth-year medical students. Attendings were students once too and recognize the hassles involved in interviewing across the country. Most will understand if you miss a day or two here and there.

Students who interview in January may have a slight advantage over those who interview earlier. Because these students' interviews occur after the holi-

TABLE 2-1. **Deciding When to Do Your Second AI**

ADVANTAGES OF DOING SECOND AI EARLY

- Offers another chance for a strong letter of recommendation (especially if third-year performance was weak)
- Strong evaluation on dean's letter a major plus
- Allows for a cushy spring schedule

ADVANTAGES OF DOING SECOND AI LATE

- Evaluation won't be included in dean's letter; more freedom to dictate learning objectives
- Tough rotations are distributed more evenly in fourth year; prevents burnout

days, committee members may be more likely to remember their applications and to push for them during highly charged ranking sessions. In addition, it may be hard for you to remember the specifics of a program you visited in December when making your rank-order list (ROL) in February. If you interview early, consider revisiting programs that you plan to rank highly both to refresh your memory and to reiterate your interest to the selection committee.

If you plan to hit many programs in the Northeast or upper Midwest, however, January may be a bad month because of winter traveling conditions. During the first week of January, one of us got stranded at a subway stop in a blizzard while visiting a program in Cleveland. A half-hour trip from the airport to the university thus turned into a two-and-a-half-hour ordeal. In January 1999, many students got caught in a Chicago blizzard for three days and missed subsequent interviews. The events of September 11 have delayed travel at every level in the airport, from check-in to landing. So allow extra time during snow season for visiting programs in these areas.

As a final note, try to schedule some fun into each interview trip; otherwise the burden of schlepping from one city to the next gets overwhelming. See that big arch in St. Louis, eat some chowdah in Boston, and try and make it to the beach in January in San Diego! In addition to having a good time, you will learn what each city is like at its best, which will help you when you return home to make ROL-related decisions.

Travel takes time. Snow, security check-ins, and bad luck can all ruin your trip. Arriving early can save it!

SHOULD I STICK AROUND MY SCHOOL ON MATCH DAY?

The month featuring Match Day (March for most applicants) is generally not a good time to be vacationing or doing electives outside the country. A certain percentage of U.S. medical students and international medical graduates (IMGs) will not be placed on Match Day and will have to enter the Scramble. If you do not match and have to enter the Scramble or if there is a problem with your ROL, you'll need to be in close communication with your dean and your adviser, either in person or by phone. This is especially true if you are trying to match in a competitive specialty. So if you feel the need to flee, try to choose another time. If you must be out of the country, make contingency plans with your dean and adviser, and get access to a fax machine. The WebROLIC system will allow you to find out if and where you matched via the Internet—but keep in mind that many students will be logging in on Match Day, and it may be easier to call your dean's office.

Play it safe: Try to be in the country on Match Day.

SHOULD I DO AUDITION ROTATIONS?

Early in the fourth year, many students do audition rotations (away rotations or externships) at other schools in their target specialties either to find out more about a specific program or to improve their chances of entering that program. Be careful. An away rotation is a two-edged sword—you can stumble as well as shine. Remember that you will probably be compared with medical students at that institution who are already familiar with the hospital environment and its faculty.

Away subinternships can hurt as much as they help.

On the positive side, many programs will grant visiting students a "courtesy interview" at the end of an audition rotation. In fact, some programs in certain competitive specialties, such as orthopedic surgery or emergency medicine, take only "known quantities"—students who have done rotations on site.

For the rest of you, consider doing away rotations only if you are aiming for a long-shot program in which you would not otherwise have a chance. If people from your medical school have matched at the program you are considering, keep in mind that the program likely has a positive impression of your medical school, so an away rotation may actually diminish your candidacy. If no one from your school has ever matched at that program, an audition rotation may give you that "foot in the door" as long as you do an excellent job. In evaluating the potential benefits of an audition rotation, you must size up whether you come across better in person or on paper. If you simply want to find out more about a program at a specific institution, consider doing an away rotation there, but not in your target specialty (e.g., emergency medicine at an institution whose surgery program interests you). Otherwise, you risk exposing yourself to unnecessary scrutiny.

WHAT ABOUT OTHER ELECTIVES?

Use the fourth year to learn new things and have fun, not to reproduce your internship.

Your fourth year is a fantastic opportunity to fulfill your intellectual and personal curiosity by sampling all that medicine has to offer. Don't waste it! Although it's wise to take an elective or two that will prepare you for internship (see Table 2-2), do not try to duplicate your internship during your fourth year—you'll get more than enough experience during your residency training. In addition, you might consider taking some electives that may not be available to you again. Your career adviser should have some good suggestions for fourth-year electives, as will students in the class ahead of you. Some to consider might be to travel abroad and do an international elective. You may never see those strange parasitic diseases you learned so much about in the second year here in the United States, but they are out there! Research electives can also give you insight into the direction your field is going. This might be interesting for you on a personal level and will provide excellent conversation for those low points in the interview!

WHEN SHOULD I SCHEDULE VACATION?

A national meeting can be fun, but don't go too far out of your way to attend.

Don't forget to take time for yourself. Some students take a light rotation during September of their fourth year or take two weeks off during that period so that they can attend to residency applications. Remember that once residency starts, you will be limited to two to five weeks of vacation per year—and you can probably forget holidays such as Christmas, Hanukkah, and Thanksgiving.

Your school may finance a trip to a national meeting if you present.

Consider spending part of your vacation at a major national meeting in one or two of your top specialty choices either late in your third year or early in your fourth year, especially if the meeting is nearby or if your adviser is planning to go. A list of national meetings is published regularly in *JAMA* as well as on specialty organization Web sites (see Table 2-3). Most of these conferences have special reduced registration rates for medical students. Some students submit abstracts based on clinical cases, which may enable them to obtain travel and registration funding from the department and/or dean's office. Your career adviser can provide more detailed information about the best ones to attend. At these meetings, you can meet the field's celebrities, find out what's hot, hear about problems and politics, scope out the turf wars, etc. You can preview programs in the specialty by looking at research posters or by listening

TABLE 2-2. Recommended Fourth-Year Electives by Specialty

SPECIALTY	RECOMMENDED ELECTIVES FOR INTERNSHIP	RELATED ELECTIVES
Anesthesiology	Surgical ICU	Radiology, emergency medicine, medical ethics
Dermatology	Infectious disease, medicine subinternship, pathology	Emergency medicine, ophthalmology, pediatric subinternship
Emergency medicine	ICU, radiology, gynecology, trauma surgery	Cardiology, dermatology, psychiatry crisis center, toxicology
Family practice	Cardiology, emergency medicine, gastroenterology, orthopedics	Dermatology, ophthalmology, overseas elective, radiology, sports medicine
Internal medicine	Cardiology, emergency medicine, infectious disease, pulmonary	Dermatology, orthopedics, OB/GYN, otolaryngology, overseas elective
Neurology	Psychiatry subinternship, radiology, geriatrics	Neurosurgery, emergency medicine
Obstetrics and gynecology	Maternal/fetal medicine, pediatrics, surgery subinternship, urology	Emergency medicine, family practice, endocrinology
Orthopedics	Emergency medicine, trauma surgery	ICU, rheumatology, radiology, sports medicine
Otolaryngology	Emergency medicine, neurology, surgery subinternship	Dermatology, pulmonary medicine
Ophthalmology	Emergency medicine, neurology	Dermatology, medicine consult
Pathology	Clinical anatomy, radiology	Laboratory medicine, infectious disease, hematology
Pediatrics	Emergency medicine, dermatology, pediatric infectious disease, pediatric intensive care medicine	Child psychiatry, medicine consult, radiology, pediatric surgery
Psychiatry	Endocrinology, neurology subinternship, medicine consult	Emergency medicine, toxicology, substance abuse
Radiology	Clinical anatomy, anatomic pathology	Informatics, orthopedics, emergency medicine
Surgery	Emergency medicine, ICU, trauma surgery, clinical anatomy	Medicine consult, surgical pathology, anesthesiology

SETTING UP THE FOURTH YEAR

TABLE 2-3. Partial List of Specialty Organizations

SETTING UP THE FOURTH YEAR

SPECIALTY	ORGANIZATION/CONTACT INFORMATION	WEB SITE
General	American Medical Women's Association (AMWA) 801 North Fairfax Street, Suite 400 Alexandria, VA 22314 (703) 838-0500 Fax: (703) 549-3864	www.amwa-doc.org
	American Medical Association (AMA) 515 North State Street Chicago, IL 60610 (312) 464-5000	www.ama-assn.org
	American Medical Student Association (AMSA) 1902 Association Drive Reston, VA 20191 (703) 620-6600 Fax: (703) 620-5873	www.amsa.org
Anesthesiology	American Society of Anesthesiologists (ASA) 520 North Northwest Highway Park Ridge, IL 60068 (847) 825-5586 Fax: (847) 825-1692	www.asahq.org
Dermatology	American Academy of Dermatology (AAD) P.O. Box 4014 Schaumberg, IL 60168-4014 (847) 330-0230, ext. 365 Fax: (847) 330-0050	www.aad.org
Emergency medicine	American College of Emergency Physicians (ACEP) P.O. Box 619911 Dallas, TX 75261-9911 (972) 550-0911 or (800) 798-1822 Fax: (972) 580-2816	www.acep.org
	Society for Academic Emergency Medicine (SAEM) 901 North Washington Avenue Lansing, MI 48906-5137 (517) 485-5484 Fax: (517) 485-0801	www.saem.org
	American Academy of Emergency Medicine (AAEM) 555 East Wells Street, Suite 1100 Milwaukee, WI 53202 (800) 884-2236 Fax: (414) 276-3349	www.aaem.org

TABLE 2-3. Partial List of Specialty Organizations (continued)

SPECIALTY	ORGANIZATION/CONTACT INFORMATION	WEB SITE
	Emergency Medicine Residents' Association (EMRA) 1125 Executive Circle Dallas, TX 75261-9911 (972) 550-0920 or (800) 798-1822 Fax: (972) 580-2829	www.emra.org
Family practice	American Academy of Family Physicians (AAFP) 11400 Tomahawk Creek Parkway Leawood, KS 66211-2672 (913) 906-6000, ext. 5224, or (800) 274-2237, ext. 5224	www.aafp.org
Internal medicine	American College of Physicians (ACP) 190 North Independence Mall West Philadelphia, PA 19106-1572 (215) 351-2600 or (800) 523-1546, ext. 2600	www.acponline.org
	American College of Preventive Medicine (ACPM) 1307 New York Avenue, N.W., Suite 200 Washington, D.C. 20005 (202) 466-2044 Fax: (202) 466-2662	www.acpm.org
	American Geriatrics Society (AGS) Empire State Building 350 Fifth Avenue, Suite 801 New York, NY 10118 (212) 308-1414 Fax: (212) 832-8646	www.americangeriatrics.org
Neurology	American Academy of Neurology (AAN) 1080 Montreal Avenue St. Paul, MN 55116 (651) 695-2717 or (800) 879-1960 Fax: (651) 695-2791	www.aan.com
Neurosurgery	American Association of Neurological Surgeons (AANS) 5550 Meadowbrook Drive Rolling Meadows, IL 60008 (847) 378-0500 or (888) 566-2267 Fax: (847) 378-0600	www.aans.org
Obstetrics and gynecology	American College of Obstetricians and Gynecologists (ACOG) 409 12th Street, S.W. P.O. Box 96920 Washington, D.C. 20090-6920 (202) 638-5577	www.acog.org

SETTING UP THE FOURTH YEAR

TABLE 2-3. Partial List of Specialty Organizations (continued)

SPECIALTY	ORGANIZATION/CONTACT INFORMATION	WEB SITE
Ophthalmology	American Academy of Ophthalmology (AAO) P.O. Box 7424 San Francisco, CA 94120-7424 (415) 561-8500 Fax: (415) 561-8533	www.aao.org
Orthopedics	American Academy of Orthopaedic Surgeons (AAOS) 6300 North River Road Rosemont, IL 60018-4262 (847) 823-7186 Fax: (847) 843-8125	www.aaos.org
Otolaryngology	American Academy of Otolaryngology— Head and Neck Surgery (AAO-HNS) One Prince Street Alexandria, VA 22314 (703) 836-4444	www.entnet.org
Pathology	College of American Pathologists (CAP) 325 Waukegan Road Northfield, IL 60093 (800) 323-4040 or (847) 832-7000 Fax: (847) 832-8000	www.cap.org
	American Society for Clinical Pathology (ASCP) 2100 West Harrison Street Chicago, IL 60612-3798 (312) 738-1336 or (800) 621-4142 Fax: (312) 738-1619	www.ascp.org
Pediatrics	American Academy of Pediatrics (AAP) 141 Northwest Point Boulevard Elk Grove Village, IL 60007 (847) 434-4000 Fax: (847) 434-8000	www.aap.org
Physical medicine and rehabilitation	American Academy of Physical Medicine and Rehabilitation (AAPM&R) 330 North Wabash Avenue, Suite 2500 Chicago, IL 60611-7617 (312) 464-9700 Fax: (312) 464-0227	www.aapmr.org
Psychiatry	American Psychiatric Association (APA) 1000 Wilson Boulevard, Suite 1825 Arlington, VA 22209-3901 (703) 907-7300	www.psych.org

TABLE 2-3. Partial List of Specialty Organizations (continued)

SPECIALTY	ORGANIZATION/CONTACT INFORMATION	WEB SITE
	American Academy of Child and Adolescent Psychiatry (AACAP) 3615 Wisconsin Avenue, N.W. Washington, D.C. 20016 (202) 966-7300 Fax: (202) 966-2891	www.aacap.org
Radiology	American College of Radiology (ACR) 1891 Preston White Drive Reston, VA 20191-4397 (703) 648-8900 or (800) ACR-LINE	www.acr.org
	Radiological Society of North America (RSNA) 820 Jorie Boulevard Oak Brook, IL 60523-2251 (630) 571-2670 or (800) 381-6660 Fax: (630) 571-7837	www.rsna.org
Radiation oncology	American College of Radiation Oncology (ACRO) 5272 River Road Bethesda, MD 20816 (301) 718-6515 Fax: (301) 656-0989	www.acro.org
	American Society for Therapeutic Radiology and Oncology (ASTRO) 12500 Fair Lakes Circle, Suite 375 Fairfax, VA 22033-3882 (800) 962-7876 or (703) 502-1550 Fax: (703) 502-7852	www.astro.org
Surgery	American College of Surgeons (ACS) 633 North Saint Clair Street Chicago, IL 60611 (312) 202-5000 or (800) 621-4111 Fax: (312) 202-5001	www.facs.org
	American College of Chest Physicians (ACCP) 3300 Dundee Road Northbrook, IL 60062 (847) 498-1400 or (800) 343-2227 Fax: (847) 498-5460	www.chestnet.org
	American Society of Colon and Rectal Surgeons (ASCRS) 85 West Algonquin Road, Suite 550 Arlington Heights, IL 60005 (847) 290-9184 Fax: (847) 290-9203	www.fascrs.org

SETTING UP THE FOURTH YEAR

TABLE 2-3. Partial List of Specialty Organizations (continued)

SPECIALTY	ORGANIZATION/CONTACT INFORMATION	WEB SITE
Urology	American Urological Association (AUA) 1000 Corporate Boulevard Linthicum, MD 21090 (866) RING-AUA (866-746-4282) Fax: (410) 689-3800	www.auanet.org

to scheduled faculty talks. Spending time at a major meeting will provide you with valuable insights and perspectives and can also make you a more knowledgeable and interesting candidate during interviews.

You may want to take one of two approaches to vacation during the fourth year. Those students applying to ten or more programs should probably use at least some of their vacation time for interviews in January and December as described above. Alternatively, those students who are applying to fewer programs might want to do all their interviews "on the fly" during clinical rotations in the fourth year. This will allow you to finish your fourth-year requirements and take a sizable (two-month) vacation, right after Match Day!

References

American Academy of Child and Adolescent Psychiatry Web site (www. aacap.org).
American Academy of Dermatology Web site (www.aad.org).
American Academy of Emergency Medicine Web site (www.aaem.org).
American Academy of Family Physicians Web site (www.aafp.org).
American Academy of Neurology Web site (www.aan.com).
American Academy of Ophthalmology Web site (www.aao.org).
American Academy of Orthopaedic Surgeons Web site (www.aaos.org).
American Academy of Otolaryngology—Head and Neck Surgery Web site (www.entnet.org).
American Academy of Pediatrics Web site (www.aap.org).
American Academy of Physical Medicine and Rehabilitation Web site (www.aapmr.org).
American Association of Neurological Surgeons Web site (www.aans.org).
American College of Chest Physicians Web site (www.chestnet.org).
American College of Emergency Physicians Web site (www.acep.org).
American College of Obstetricians and Gynecologists Web site (www.acog.org).
American College of Physicians Web site (www.acponline.org).
American College of Preventive Medicine Web site (www.acpm.org).
American College of Radiation Oncology Web site (www.acro.org).
American College of Radiology Web site (www.acr.org).
American College of Surgeons Web site (www.facs.org).
American Geriatrics Society Web site (www.americangeriatrics.org).
American Medical Association Web site (www.ama-assn.org).
American Medical Student Association Web site (www.amsa.org).
American Medical Women's Association Web site (www.amwa-doc.org).
American Psychiatric Association Web site (www.psych.org).
American Society for Therapeutic Radiology and Oncology Web site (www.astro.org).
American Society of Anesthesiologists Web site (www.asahq.org).
American Society of Colon and Rectal Surgeons Web site (www.fascrs.org).
American Society for Clinical Pathology Web site (www.ascp.org).
American Urological Association Web site (www.auanet.org).
College of American Pathologists Web site (www.cap.org).
Emergency Medicine Residents' Association Web site (www.emra.org).

Fellowship and Residency Electronic Interactive Database (FREIDA) American Medical Association Web site (www.ama-assn.org/ama/pub/category/2997.html).

National Resident Matching Program Web site (www.nrmp.org).

Radiological Society of North America Web site (www.rsna.org).

Reference directories. *JAMA* 273(21):1652, 1995.

Society for Academic Emergency Medicine Web site (www.saem.org).

Wagoner NE, Suriano R, Stoner JA. Factors used by program directors to select residents. *J Med Educ* 61(1):10–21, 1986.

Choosing and Matching in Your Specialty

Choosing a specialty may be one of the most difficult decisions a student encounters during medical school. Ironically, this life decision comes at an early time in the medical experience. Although some students confidently know their specialty calling after limited clinical exposure during the third year, many students are still attracted to more than one specialty. The summer months after the third year provide a crucial time to further explore career options with electives and subinternships. Rotations at an away site during this time may provide an important new perspective by allowing the student to work with different faculty members.

As the end of summer approaches, students should have finalized their decision about the type of residency they wish to pursue. Any lingering indecision could have a negative impact on the application process that begins in September. Before the fall of their senior year, students will be expected to write personal statements that reflect their commitment to a particular area, choose faculty to write letters of recommendation (based in part on career choice), and begin to prepare for interviews.

The beginning of the fourth year, when third-year experiences are still clear in students' minds, is the best time to choose a career and residency type. There are fewer exams and call nights, leaving students ample time to contemplate this critical decision. Schedules are also flexible at this time, allowing students to choose experiences that can aid in decision making. Nonetheless, some students need additional time to explore their options. There are two major reasons students fail to make this important decision by the fall of the year:

1. One or more specialties appear very attractive, making it difficult for students to choose among several opportunities; or
2. No single career choice stands out above the others.

WEIGHING YOUR OPTIONS

It may be of some use for undecided students to review what is currently known about student specialty choices in general:

- Students who experience ambulatory care electives and clerkships are more likely to select a primary care specialty.
- Students who are exposed to high-tech experiences and research in their third and fourth years are inclined to switch from primary care to university-based surgical specialties.
- Students who choose primary care specialties are more likely to be highly influenced by mentors than are those who opt for high-tech specialties.
- Some personality traits tend to correlate with specialty choice. Myers-Briggs personality traits of feeling and introversion tend to correlate with primary care fields. Surgical specialties are favored by those classified as extroverted and "thinking." However, neither students going into primary care nor those entering surgery are a homogeneous group.
- Recent graduates may be increasingly concerned about issues of lifestyle, time with family, and level of stress, all of which explain the trend away from surgery as a specialty choice.
- Students who have gone through a process such as the Glaxo Pathway Evaluation Program find that process useful and often refer back to its results to confirm their final decision.

- Several studies have reported that over time, approximately 25% of physicians change their specialty choice. Financial and lifestyle issues usually underlie this rethinking process. Relatively few physicians seem to regret their choice because they lacked challenge.

Reading current literature and data about specialty choices can be helpful, but do not let it distract you from the heart of this very personal decision. If you are undecided, it is important to ask yourself questions about your personal and professional needs. Some questions to ponder include:

- What were your original goals when you decided to become a physician? Are they still valid? If not, what has changed and why?
- What part of a physician's role do you value the most? Is it the long-standing patient relationships, the ability to immediately help others, the intellectual challenge, the prestige, or using the newest technology to help patients?
- What type of doctor-patient relationship do you find the most rewarding?
- What personal strengths do you feel you can offer to medicine? What skills (interpersonal, communication, technical, analytical, etc.) do you value most in yourself and hope to highlight during your career?
- What situations make you uncomfortable? In which types of patient encounters do you feel that you are not reaching your full potential?

In order to answer these questions, you must be honest with yourself. Only then will you be able to let your innate values, goals, and expectations guide you toward an appropriate specialty choice.

For students who have identified and explored more than one excellent career option, it is likely that they will excel in either of their choices. In addition to thinking about the questions listed above, it may also be helpful to review the categories that are commonly used in choosing a specialty and reorder their importance. Such categories usually include:

- Personal satisfaction
- Family issues
- Prestige factor
- Salary
- Working conditions

Again, by honestly looking at one's own values, goals, and expectations, the appropriate specialty choice will become more obvious. Students may, in addition, find it useful to review FREIDA online physician workforce information to compare hours, salaries, and job satisfaction data from among the various specialties. Other helpful references for students who need more help are listed at the end of the chapter.

Family and lifestyle are increasingly critical factors.

WHAT IF I STILL CAN'T DECIDE?

For students who remain undecided at the "last hour," emphasis on personal satisfaction is key. Such students should ask the question "What would make me most happy?" or "What would give me the most job satisfaction?" Most physicians would agree that enjoying the day-to-day work of the profession is critical to success and that all other considerations are secondary. So when time has run out and a decision must be made in order for the matching process to proceed, you should determine what you most enjoy doing and then go for it! It may be that excessive concerns about the opinion of a relative or spouse, an adviser's assessment of a particular field, or workload or salary issues are precisely what led to your indecision in the first place. If you are content with what you are doing, factors such as salary, workload, and prestige will usually become secondary.

For students who cannot arrive at any good residency choice, the problem is much more significant. The profession of medicine offers an incredible variety of opportunities, so students should have found an attractive choice by the fall of their senior year. If the fall of your senior year has arrived and you still have no attractive specialty choice in sight, good counseling is imperative. Meetings with your senior adviser and associate dean of students should be scheduled immediately if they have not already taken place.

It should be noted, however, that few educators will recommend that students take a year away from medicine, since such a hiatus may lead students to stray from their career choice despite the considerable investment they have already made in both time and effort. One solid exception to this rule may be a year dedicated to medical research for students who are interested in pursuing an academic career or are preparing for a competitive residency. Many have found that a productive research year can significantly bolster CVs and improve their ability to compete for these residency positions. There are also other options for the year following the completion of medical school, including a transitional year or a preliminary-year residency.

Transitional year. A transitional year, while popular in the past, is usually not seen to be beneficial for specialty decision making. A few programs may be designed for this purpose, but most are so rigorous that they may only frustrate students who could not choose a specialty under the much more favorable circumstances of their senior year. A transitional program will usually result in essentially two years of internship—a formidable task for even the most enthusiastic student. Little additional information about the core specialties is likely to be obtained.

Preliminary year. A preliminary year may be a better option than a transitional year for the undecided student. The preliminary year of medicine or surgery can be used to guide a student's choice of specialty, particularly if he or she is leaning toward either medicine or surgery. A preliminary year will also eliminate the need to repeat an internship and may be used as a prerequisite for such fields as radiology, anesthesiology, radiation oncology, and rehabilitation medicine. Some programs will offer four months of elective time that may be used to obtain additional experiences and hence facilitate the decision-making process. A preliminary year in one's own medical school is usually advisable if the year is needed for specialty decision making. Some preliminary program directors will enthusiastically support tailoring the year for this purpose. The preliminary year differs from a categorical position in that a preliminary year is a one-year position meant for people going into a specialty (anesthesia, radiology, etc.) that requires one year of another specialty first, or for people who are undecided or unmatched in the specialty of their choice. It counts toward one's residency training (versus the transitional year, which does not) in terms of board-exam eligibility, but the program is under no obligation to grant the next year of training. A categorical position is one in surgery, medicine, or any other specialty that ensures one a position for the full time course of his or her training.

A preliminary or transitional year can buy more time to decide.

Each specialty calls for a different approach toward preparing a successful application and interview. For example, psychiatry residency directors expect and appreciate in-depth personal statements with a thorough exploration of an applicant's background and motives for entering the specialty. Other specialties, such as orthopedics and neurosurgery, are heavily influenced by audition rotations.

In this chapter, we briefly profile selected specialties. (See Table 4-1 for factors considered by medical students in choosing a specialty.) We have organized the information and advice for each specialty under the following headings:

- **Overview:** The specialty in terms of recent trends in the medical career market.
- **Match Numbers:** An analysis of recent Match results.
- **Application Tips:** Advice and guidance for the application process specific to each specialty.
- **Interview Tips:** Advice and guidance for the interview visit specific to that specialty.
- **For More Info:** A collection of essential career and residency application resources for each specialty.

The **Overview,** a brief description of the specialty itself as well as a glance at its socioeconomic trends, summarizes student, resident, and faculty observations. It is *not* intended as a basis for the complex and critical process of specialty selection. For more in-depth information about the specialty, consult the following resources:

- Faculty and house staff in the field.
- Brochures from the academic or certifying society in the field (listed under "For More Info").
- The Glaxo Pathway Evaluation Program, a free half-day seminar sometimes offered by the dean's office that helps you match your interests to different specialties. These seminars feature the *Glaxo Medical Specialties Survey* (1991), a catalog of medical specialties and subspecialties that includes descriptions, practitioner profiles, and anecdotal "picks and pans." Contact your student affairs office for details.
- Iserson KV, *Iserson's Getting into a Residency*, 5th ed., Tucson, AZ: Galen Press, 2000.

ANESTHESIOLOGY

Factors attracting students to careers in anesthesiology include brief but positive doctor-patient relationships, above-average income (see Figure 4-1D), and immediate results. Anesthesiologists play an integral part in the practice of medicine, including the presurgical center, operating room, postanesthesia care unit, ICU, and pain management center, as well as throughout the hospital. The field offers significant respect and intellectual stimulation and tends to involve relatively predictable hours. It is a hospital-based specialty with frequent night calls. Most recent graduates find good job opportunities. Many residency program graduates go on to fellowship training in areas such as critical care and pain management.

Some students have difficulty choosing among careers that they believe offer critical lifestyle advantages. When a student chooses a list of fields such as radiology, emergency medicine, anesthesiology, and radiation oncology, the problem may lie in priorities. These fields have little in common and may not really provide the lifestyle advantage that students presume them to have. Counseling from program directors in these fields is the most appropriate course of action in such cases.

In some cases, students may be committed to a primary care field but have trouble deciding among the primary care specialties. A student attempting to choose between medicine and family medicine, for example, might compare the diversity of experiences in family medicine to the more frequent diagnostic challenges and fellowship opportunities found in medicine. Some students with an interest in obstetrics and primary care may seek to find out more about opportunities to practice obstetrics within the field of family medicine. Similarly, the choice between family medicine and medicine-pediatrics may be governed by a student's interest in obstetrics or by his or her willingness to study for two board exams and keep up with the literature in two separate fields.

For other students, career preferences may meet up with the harsh realities of competition. For example, a student may realize in the fall of senior year that he or she is highly unlikely to match in programs such as dermatology, orthopedics, or ophthalmology. Such students should seek good counseling, not only to optimize their chances of selection but also to help them choose from among alternative fields. This choice of alternatives should be based on their attraction to the competitive fields.

Often, students who are attracted to a specialty area may be held back by self-doubt. Perhaps they lean toward orthopedics but fear that they are not physically strong enough, want to enter internal medicine but fear they are not smart enough, or are attracted to surgery but fear they are not tough enough. Students in this "indecision mode" are usually advised to proceed as if their concerns did not exist. Such fears are usually easy to overcome and should not deter students from what they really want to do.

When time has run out and a career decision must be made, take solace in knowing that all the facts and experiences you need are already in your mind. Choose the area of medicine that has appealed to you most! Do not delay decision making. Do not carve out another year of indecision. Do not try to find someone to make the choice for you. Remember why you wanted to become a physician in the first place. If you have lost confidence in yourself with exposure to so many other talented colleagues, reclaim that confidence. The right amount of confidence and passion will lead you to the right decision.

References

Ellsbury KE, Carline JD, Irby DM, Stritter FT. Influence of third-year clerkship on medical student specialty choice. *Adv Health Sci Educ Theory Pract* 3(3):177–186, 1998.

Gelfand DV, Podnos YD, Wilson SE, Cooke J, Williams RA. Choosing general surgery: insights into career choices of current medical students. *Arch Surg* 137(8):941–945, 2002.

Pugno PA, McPherson DS, Schmittling GT, Kahn NB. Results of the National Resident Matching Program: family practice. *Fam Med* 34(8):584–591, 2002.

TABLE 4-1. Most Influential Factors Determining Specialty Choice

Type and range of patient problems encountered

Appropriateness for personality

Opportunity to make a difference in people's lives

Desire to help people

Intellectual appeal of the specialty

The challenge of diagnostic problems

Diversity of diagnosis and therapy

Reed VA, Jernstedt GC, Reber ES. Understanding and improving medical student specialty choice: a synthesis of the literature using decision theory as a referent. *Teach Learn Med* 13(2):117–129, 2001.

Stearns MA, Wallick MM, Jobe AC. Senior students' evaluation of the usefulness of the Glaxo Pathway Evaluation Program. *Acad Med* 68:638–640, 1993.

Stillwell NA, Wallick MM, Thal SE, Burleson JA. Myers-Briggs type and medical specialty choice: a new look at an old question. *Teach Learn Med* 12(1):14–21, 2000.

Tardiff K, Celia D, Seiferth C, Perry S. Selection and change of specialties by medical student graduates. *J Med Educ* 61:790–796, 1986.

Wallick MM, Cambre KM, Randall HM. Personality type and medical specialty choice. *J La State Med Soc* 151:463–468, 1999.

CHAPTER 4

Your Specialty and the Match

ANESTHESIOLOGY

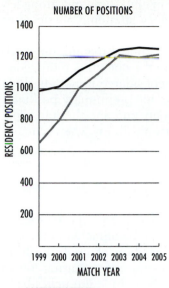

NUMBER OF POSITIONS

— POSITIONS OFFERED
— POSITIONS FILLED

A. Positions offered in anesthesiology and number filled.

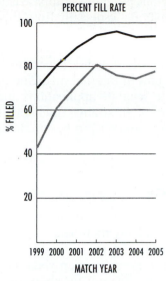

PERCENT FILL RATE

— TOTAL % FILLED
— U.S. % FILLED

B. Percentage of anesthesiology positions filled on Match Day.

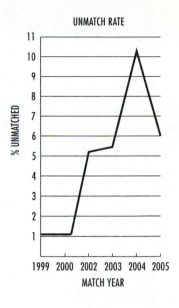

UNMATCH RATE

C. Percentage of U.S. seniors unmatched in anesthesiology on Match Day.

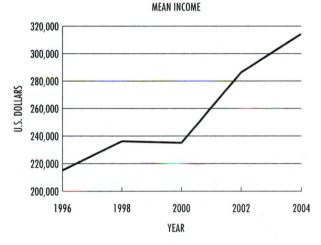

MEAN INCOME

D. Mean income of anesthesiologists in U.S. dollars.

FIGURES 4-1A–D

Match Numbers

In 2005, there were 463 PGY-1 positions and 820 PGY-2 positions offered in anesthesiology (see Figure 4-1A). The overall fill rate remained steady at approximately 95% from 2002 to 2005, up from 80% in 2000 and 35% in 1996 (see Figures 4-1B and C). The percentage of positions filled by U.S. medical graduates has also risen gradually, from a low 17.3% in 1996 to 54.5% in 2000 to 70% in 2005. The number of positions offered by anesthesiology programs steadily increased from 1998 to 2004.

Application Tips

Most prestigious programs emphasize good grades in clerkships and strong letters of evaluation—especially from the anesthesiology attending physician or the head of the anesthesiology department. Good grades in physiology and pharmacology might be especially appealing to some program directors. Given that anesthesiologists act as the "internists" in the operating room, good clerkship grades in internal medicine may also be considered important. Plan to coordinate separate applications and interviews for preliminary positions. Hospitals can often arrange interviews for preliminary and anesthesiology positions on the same day, so be sure to ask about this possibility when scheduling interviews.

Interview Tips

Interviews are usually conducted in December and January. Many program directors and faculty members feel that students might be attracted to the specialty for the wrong reasons—e.g., a student's perception of lifestyle advantages. Anesthesiologists often view their job as stressful and requiring lots of night calls. Valid reasons for choosing anesthesiology include the field's basic science underpinning, interest in both surgery and medicine, and participation on a highly sophisticated team.

For More Info . . .

- *American Society of Anesthesiologists Information Packet.* This free career information packet includes general articles (of marginal value) on the specialty itself, a directory of anesthesiology training programs as listed in the *Graduate Medical Education Directory*, and a directory of fellowships for specialized training in pain management. The packet can be obtained by contacting:

  American Society of Anesthesiologists (ASA)
  520 North Northwest Highway
  Park Ridge, IL 60068
  (847) 825-5586
  www.asahq.org

- Global Anesthesiology Server Network
  www.gasnet.org

DERMATOLOGY

Dermatologists in the United States today enjoy some of the most pleasant demographics of any specialty. They work the lowest number of hours per week while getting paid more than any other nonsurgical specialty. Mean incomes for dermatologists currently hover around $200,000. They also have a typically healthy patient population and are to a large extent immune to the increasing number of HMO-dictated regulations, as many patient visits are paid for out-of-pocket.

However, the field suffers from a poor distribution of physicians; although there are openings available in smaller communities and rural areas, most urban centers are saturated. Moreover, in today's managed-care environment, an increasing number of relatively routine and mild skin diseases are being treated by primary care physicians. As a result, more attention is being paid to the diagnosis of oncologic diseases, surgical procedures, and cosmetic treatments not covered by managed-care contracts.

Training in dermatology requires one year of internship followed by three years of residency. A preliminary medicine year is preferable, but any training involving clinical patient care, such as surgery or transitional medicine, may be acceptable. Be sure to check with individual programs to see which type of preliminary-year training they will accept. A small number of programs offer dermatology residency positions combined with a preliminary year in internal medicine. (These are listed as categorical positions in ERAS.) In 2005, 28 of these positions were offered. Advanced positions require that applicants secure their own preliminary year. Residency training includes diagnostic and therapeutic procedures, both medical and surgical, with the emphasis varying according to the particular program.

Match Numbers

Dermatology continues to be one of the most difficult specialties in which to match. In 2002, 16% of U.S. seniors who applied in dermatology failed to match (see Figure 4-2C). In the same time period, the number of positions in dermatology programs has slowly continued to increase, up from 275 positions in 2002 to 316 positions in 2005 (see Figure 4-2A). Dermatology continues to be one of the most competitive specialties, with nearly 100% of positions filled each year, 77% of which were filled by U.S. medical students in 2005 (see Figure 4-2B). These intimidating numbers show no signs of abating in the near future.

DERMATOLOGY

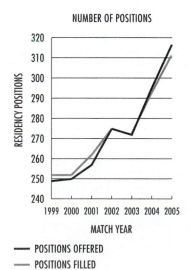

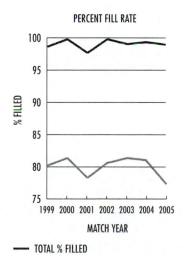

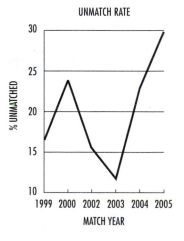

A. Positions offered in dermatology and number filled.

B. Percentage of dermatology positions filled on Match Day.

C. Percentage of U.S. seniors unmatched in dermatology on Match Day.

FIGURES 4-2A–C

A track record in dermatology research is considered a big plus.

Application Tips

Given the competitive nature of dermatology, all aspects of the residency application are important. Dermatology programs screen applicants intensively before offering interviews to prospective residents. Many use AΩA status, at least three honors in clinical rotations, high board scores, and a top-notch dean's letter as preliminary considerations. Competitive programs often use the USMLE Step 1 score to screen applications, and research in dermatology is highly recommended. A glowing evaluation in the dermatology subinternship and supportive letters of recommendation are vital as well. Given the competitive nature of the specialty, however, applicants need to demonstrate more than just academic excellence. Perhaps the most important aspect of the application in this field is numbers. All applicants, regardless of their CV, should apply to, interview at, and rank as many programs as they can (without violating the two rules of ranking outlined in Chapter 12). In 2005, there were 945 applicants (709 U.S. graduates and 236 IMGs) for dematology. On average, each applicant applied to 38 programs in 2005. Be prepared to spend more than the national average on application and travel expenses.

Interview Tips

Be prepared to wait; most programs don't begin offering interviews until around Thanksgiving. Many interview dates will be during the months of December ("early" interviews), January, and February. Dermatology applicants have several things in common: stellar board scores, shining letters of recommendation, and impressive research experience. Therefore, program directors rely heavily on interviews to cull the field of many superb applicants down to those few who will be ranked. Dermatology programs usually offer interviews to only 10–15% of their applicants. Many conduct multiple interviews per day (up to 12 to 15 interviews), each lasting anywhere from 8 to 30 minutes, so be prepared for a lot of questioning. Depending on the program, interviews may be conducted by individual faculty members or by a panel consisting of three or more interviewers. Interviews are designed to measure applicants' interest in the specialty; to gauge the potential of each to contribute to the field; and to find out whether applicants would get along with other people in the department. Applicants are rarely pimped but will be expected to discuss any prior research or involvement in dermatology both intelligently and in detail.

For More Info . . .

- *American Academy of Dermatology Web site.* This site includes a mind-numbing description of accredited dermatology training programs along with a list of dermatology programs worldwide and of dermatology fellowships in North America. The information can be obtained by visiting:

  www.aad.org/professionals/residents/default.htm.

References

Rubenstein DS, Blauvelt A, Chen SC, Darling TN. The future of academic dermatology in the United States: report on the resident retreat for future physician-scientists, June 15–17, 2001. *J Am Acad Dermatol* 47(2):300–303, 2002.

Todd MM, Miller JJ, Ammirati CT. Dermatologic surgery training in residency. *Dermatol Surg* 28(7):547–549, 2002.

Emergency medicine (EM) has enjoyed considerable growth over the past few years, and with good reason. Relatively abundant free time, high pay (see Figure 4-3D), and the ability to integrate medicine with surgical procedures all add to this field's appeal. Fellowships are easily obtained for those who seek further training. Postresidency academic pursuits and fellowships can range from the exotic (international health, disaster/rescue medicine, and diving medicine) to the more commonplace (ultrasound, pediatrics, toxicology). EM is one of the only specialties in which a graduating resident may have a chance at an attending position straight out of residency, but these positions are becoming increasingly rare.

Over the past ten years, a number of hospitals and academic centers have added EM departments to their services, and many of these departments house residencies. Historically, EM is infamous for a high burnout rate. However, it is the youngest board-certified specialty (primary board status was not granted until 1989), so it is difficult to determine whether physicians who were recently trained in EM will show the same burnout rate in future years. It goes without saying that the ER can be stressful and that night shifts can drag on, but the EM resident's mantra is that he or she can always go home at the end of the day.

Residency programs in EM are unique in that they require either three or four years of total training. There has been much talk in the past about standardizing the amount of training required, but this has yet to materialize. In most cases, the internship year is integrated with the main EM training. For nonintegrated programs, a separate internship in medicine, surgery, or transitional medicine is required (although you do not have to do this at the same hospital). Obviously, this extra year can have a significant impact on an applicant's choice for training. If you are considering a three-year program, make sure that program offers the number of patients and level of acuity you'll need to acquire an adequate education in the three-year period.

The bulk of EM training time is spent in emergency rooms, learning resuscitation techniques, and treating both medical and trauma-related illnesses. However, residents also rotate through specialties such as medicine, pediatrics, OB/GYN, surgery, anesthesiology, and orthopedic surgery so that they can acquire a well-rounded knowledge and develop an eye for common emergencies in these fields. Different programs place "off-service" rotations in different years throughout the residency. Once you have interviewed at various programs, several factors will determine which programs you will rank more favorably. A recent study of residents just completing the EM match process within the last year or two revealed that the top five factors that they considered when choosing a program included friendliness (95%), environment (87%), perception of program during the interview day (81%), academics (76%), and location (74%).

Match Numbers

Competition for spots in EM residencies continues to intensify despite the addition of positions over the past several match years. In 1999 there were only 1063 total spots, while in 2005 that number had increased to 1332. In 2005, 1308 positions were filled, constituting a 98% fill rate (see Figures 4-3A and B). This high fill rate marks an upward trend in the number of applicants to

NUMBER OF POSITIONS

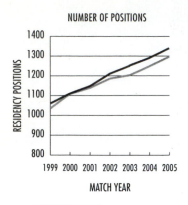

MATCH YEAR

— POSITIONS OFFERED
— POSITIONS FILLED

A. Positions offered in emergency medicine and number filled.

PERCENT FILL RATE

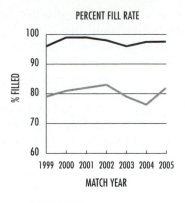

MATCH YEAR

— TOTAL % FILLED
— U.S. % FILLED

B. Percentage of emergency medicine positions filled on Match Day.

UNMATCH RATE

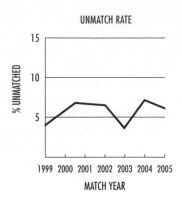

MATCH YEAR

C. Percentage of U.S. seniors unmatched in emergency medicine on Match Day.

MEAN INCOME

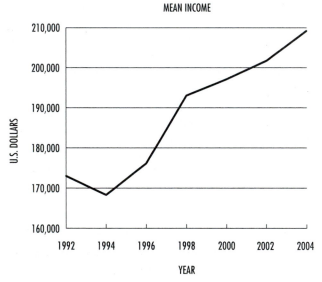

YEAR

D. Mean income of emergency medicine physicians in U.S. dollars.

FIGURES 4-3A–D

the field as EM residencies become increasingly competitive. In 2004, there were over 1500 applicants who ranked at least one EM program. In fact, 7% of all U.S. seniors who applied in EM in 2004 failed to match and had to scramble, representing an increase from previous years (see Figure 4-3C).

Application Tips

Given the competitive nature of EM, all aspects of the residency application are important. It is especially crucial to do well in an EM rotation and to ask for strong letters of recommendation from one of the attending physicians. (It would be even better to get a letter from the program director.) EM also re-

Some students have difficulty choosing among careers that they believe offer critical lifestyle advantages. When a student chooses a list of fields such as radiology, emergency medicine, anesthesiology, and radiation oncology, the problem may lie in priorities. These fields have little in common and may not really provide the lifestyle advantage that students presume them to have. Counseling from program directors in these fields is the most appropriate course of action in such cases.

In some cases, students may be committed to a primary care field but have trouble deciding among the primary care specialties. A student attempting to choose between medicine and family medicine, for example, might compare the diversity of experiences in family medicine to the more frequent diagnostic challenges and fellowship opportunities found in medicine. Some students with an interest in obstetrics and primary care may seek to find out more about opportunities to practice obstetrics within the field of family medicine. Similarly, the choice between family medicine and medicine-pediatrics may be governed by a student's interest in obstetrics or by his or her willingness to study for two board exams and keep up with the literature in two separate fields.

For other students, career preferences may meet up with the harsh realities of competition. For example, a student may realize in the fall of senior year that he or she is highly unlikely to match in programs such as dermatology, orthopedics, or ophthalmology. Such students should seek good counseling, not only to optimize their chances of selection but also to help them choose from among alternative fields. This choice of alternatives should be based on their attraction to the competitive fields.

Often, students who are attracted to a specialty area may be held back by self-doubt. Perhaps they lean toward orthopedics but fear that they are not physically strong enough, want to enter internal medicine but fear they are not smart enough, or are attracted to surgery but fear they are not tough enough. Students in this "indecision mode" are usually advised to proceed as if their concerns did not exist. Such fears are usually easy to overcome and should not deter students from what they really want to do.

When time has run out and a career decision must be made, take solace in knowing that all the facts and experiences you need are already in your mind. Choose the area of medicine that has appealed to you most! Do not delay decision making. Do not carve out another year of indecision. Do not try to find someone to make the choice for you. Remember why you wanted to become a physician in the first place. If you have lost confidence in yourself with exposure to so many other talented colleagues, reclaim that confidence. The right amount of confidence and passion will lead you to the right decision.

References

Ellsbury KE, Carline JD, Irby DM, Stritter FT. Influence of third-year clerkship on medical student specialty choice. *Adv Health Sci Educ Theory Pract* 3(3):177–186, 1998.

Gelfand DV, Podnos YD, Wilson SE, Cooke J, Williams RA. Choosing general surgery: insights into career choices of current medical students. *Arch Surg* 137(8):941–945, 2002.

Pugno PA, McPherson DS, Schmittling GT, Kahn NB. Results of the National Resident Matching Program: family practice. *Fam Med* 34(8):584–591, 2002.

Reed VA, Jernstedt GC, Reber ES. Understanding and improving medical student specialty choice: a synthesis of the literature using decision theory as a referent. *Teach Learn Med* 13(2):117–129, 2001.

Stearns MA, Wallick MM, Jobe AC. Senior students' evaluation of the usefulness of the Glaxo Pathway Evaluation Program. *Acad Med* 68:638–640, 1993.

Stillwell NA, Wallick MM, Thal SE, Burleson JA. Myers-Briggs type and medical specialty choice: a new look at an old question. *Teach Learn Med* 12(1):14–21, 2000.

Tardiff K, Celia D, Seiferth C, Perry S. Selection and change of specialties by medical student graduates. *J Med Educ* 61:790–796, 1986.

Wallick MM, Cambre KM, Randall HM. Personality type and medical specialty choice. *J La State Med Soc* 151:463–468, 1999.

CHAPTER 4

Your Specialty and the Match

Each specialty calls for a different approach toward preparing a successful application and interview. For example, psychiatry residency directors expect and appreciate in-depth personal statements with a thorough exploration of an applicant's background and motives for entering the specialty. Other specialties, such as orthopedics and neurosurgery, are heavily influenced by audition rotations.

In this chapter, we briefly profile selected specialties. (See Table 4-1 for factors considered by medical students in choosing a specialty.) We have organized the information and advice for each specialty under the following headings:

- **Overview:** The specialty in terms of recent trends in the medical career market.
- **Match Numbers:** An analysis of recent Match results.
- **Application Tips:** Advice and guidance for the application process specific to each specialty.
- **Interview Tips:** Advice and guidance for the interview visit specific to that specialty.
- **For More Info:** A collection of essential career and residency application resources for each specialty.

The **Overview,** a brief description of the specialty itself as well as a glance at its socioeconomic trends, summarizes student, resident, and faculty observations. It is *not* intended as a basis for the complex and critical process of specialty selection. For more in-depth information about the specialty, consult the following resources:

- Faculty and house staff in the field.
- Brochures from the academic or certifying society in the field (listed under "For More Info").
- The Glaxo Pathway Evaluation Program, a free half-day seminar sometimes offered by the dean's office that helps you match your interests to different specialties. These seminars feature the *Glaxo Medical Specialties Survey* (1991), a catalog of medical specialties and subspecialties that includes descriptions, practitioner profiles, and anecdotal "picks and pans." Contact your student affairs office for details.
- Iserson KV, *Iserson's Getting into a Residency*, 5th ed., Tucson, AZ: Galen Press, 2000.

TABLE 4-1. Most Influential Factors Determining Specialty Choice

Type and range of patient problems encountered
Appropriateness for personality
Opportunity to make a difference in people's lives
Desire to help people
Intellectual appeal of the specialty
The challenge of diagnostic problems
Diversity of diagnosis and therapy

ANESTHESIOLOGY

Factors attracting students to careers in anesthesiology include brief but positive doctor-patient relationships, above-average income (see Figure 4-1D), and immediate results. Anesthesiologists play an integral part in the practice of medicine, including the presurgical center, operating room, postanesthesia care unit, ICU, and pain management center, as well as throughout the hospital. The field offers significant respect and intellectual stimulation and tends to involve relatively predictable hours. It is a hospital-based specialty with frequent night calls. Most recent graduates find good job opportunities. Many residency program graduates go on to fellowship training in areas such as critical care and pain management.

ANESTHESIOLOGY

NUMBER OF POSITIONS

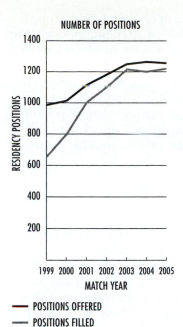

— POSITIONS OFFERED
— POSITIONS FILLED

A. Positions offered in anesthesiology and number filled.

PERCENT FILL RATE

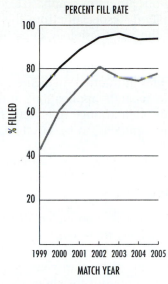

— TOTAL % FILLED
— U.S. % FILLED

B. Percentage of anesthesiology positions filled on Match Day.

UNMATCH RATE

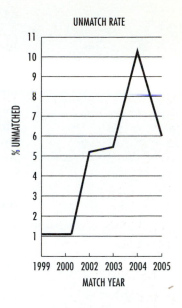

C. Percentage of U.S. seniors unmatched in anesthesiology on Match Day.

MEAN INCOME

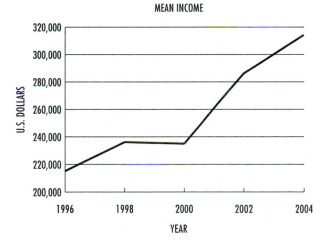

D. Mean income of anesthesiologists in U.S. dollars.

FIGURES 4-1A–D

Match Numbers

In 2005, there were 463 PGY-1 positions and 820 PGY-2 positions offered in anesthesiology (see Figure 4-1A). The overall fill rate remained steady at approximately 95% from 2002 to 2005, up from 80% in 2000 and 35% in 1996 (see Figures 4-1B and C). The percentage of positions filled by U.S. medical graduates has also risen gradually, from a low 17.3% in 1996 to 54.5% in 2000 to 70% in 2005. The number of positions offered by anesthesiology programs steadily increased from 1998 to 2004.

Application Tips

Most prestigious programs emphasize good grades in clerkships and strong letters of evaluation—especially from the anesthesiology attending physician or the head of the anesthesiology department. Good grades in physiology and pharmacology might be especially appealing to some program directors. Given that anesthesiologists act as the "internists" in the operating room, good clerkship grades in internal medicine may also be considered important. Plan to coordinate separate applications and interviews for preliminary positions. Hospitals can often arrange interviews for preliminary and anesthesiology positions on the same day, so be sure to ask about this possibility when scheduling interviews.

Interview Tips

Interviews are usually conducted in December and January. Many program directors and faculty members feel that students might be attracted to the specialty for the wrong reasons—e.g., a student's perception of lifestyle advantages. Anesthesiologists often view their job as stressful and requiring lots of night calls. Valid reasons for choosing anesthesiology include the field's basic science underpinning, interest in both surgery and medicine, and participation on a highly sophisticated team.

For More Info . . .

- *American Society of Anesthesiologists Information Packet.* This free career information packet includes general articles (of marginal value) on the specialty itself, a directory of anesthesiology training programs as listed in the *Graduate Medical Education Directory*, and a directory of fellowships for specialized training in pain management. The packet can be obtained by contacting:

    American Society of Anesthesiologists (ASA)
    520 North Northwest Highway
    Park Ridge, IL 60068
    (847) 825-5586
    www.asahq.org

- Global Anesthesiology Server Network
    www.gasnet.org

DERMATOLOGY

Dermatologists in the United States today enjoy some of the most pleasant demographics of any specialty. They work the lowest number of hours per week while getting paid more than any other nonsurgical specialty. Mean incomes for dermatologists currently hover around $200,000. They also have a typically healthy patient population and are to a large extent immune to the increasing number of HMO-dictated regulations, as many patient visits are paid for out-of-pocket.

However, the field suffers from a poor distribution of physicians; although there are openings available in smaller communities and rural areas, most urban centers are saturated. Moreover, in today's managed-care environment, an increasing number of relatively routine and mild skin diseases are being treated by primary care physicians. As a result, more attention is being paid to the diagnosis of oncologic diseases, surgical procedures, and cosmetic treatments not covered by managed-care contracts.

Training in dermatology requires one year of internship followed by three years of residency. A preliminary medicine year is preferable, but any training involving clinical patient care, such as surgery or transitional medicine, may be acceptable. Be sure to check with individual programs to see which type of preliminary-year training they will accept. A small number of programs offer dermatology residency positions combined with a preliminary year in internal medicine. (These are listed as categorical positions in ERAS.) In 2005, 28 of these positions were offered. Advanced positions require that applicants secure their own preliminary year. Residency training includes diagnostic and therapeutic procedures, both medical and surgical, with the emphasis varying according to the particular program.

Match Numbers

Dermatology continues to be one of the most difficult specialties in which to match. In 2002, 16% of U.S. seniors who applied in dermatology failed to match (see Figure 4-2C). In the same time period, the number of positions in dermatology programs has slowly continued to increase, up from 275 positions in 2002 to 316 positions in 2005 (see Figure 4-2A). Dermatology continues to be one of the most competitive specialties, with nearly 100% of positions filled each year, 77% of which were filled by U.S. medical students in 2005 (see Figure 4-2B). These intimidating numbers show no signs of abating in the near future.

DERMATOLOGY

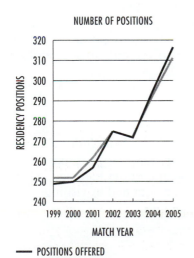

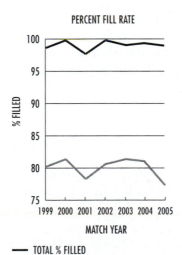

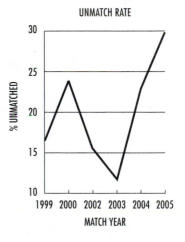

A. Positions offered in dermatology and number filled.

B. Percentage of dermatology positions filled on Match Day.

C. Percentage of U.S. seniors unmatched in dermatology on Match Day.

FIGURES 4-2A–C

Application Tips

A track record in dermatology research is considered a big plus.

Given the competitive nature of dermatology, all aspects of the residency application are important. Dermatology programs screen applicants intensively before offering interviews to prospective residents. Many use AΩA status, at least three honors in clinical rotations, high board scores, and a top-notch dean's letter as preliminary considerations. Competitive programs often use the USMLE Step 1 score to screen applications, and research in dermatology is highly recommended. A glowing evaluation in the dermatology subinternship and supportive letters of recommendation are vital as well. Given the competitive nature of the specialty, however, applicants need to demonstrate more than just academic excellence. Perhaps the most important aspect of the application in this field is numbers. All applicants, regardless of their CV, should apply to, interview at, and rank as many programs as they can (without violating the two rules of ranking outlined in Chapter 12). In 2005, there were 945 applicants (709 U.S. graduates and 236 IMGs) for dematology. On average, each applicant applied to 38 programs in 2005. Be prepared to spend more than the national average on application and travel expenses.

Interview Tips

Be prepared to wait; most programs don't begin offering interviews until around Thanksgiving. Many interview dates will be during the months of December ("early" interviews), January, and February. Dermatology applicants have several things in common: stellar board scores, shining letters of recommendation, and impressive research experience. Therefore, program directors rely heavily on interviews to cull the field of many superb applicants down to those few who will be ranked. Dermatology programs usually offer interviews to only 10–15% of their applicants. Many conduct multiple interviews per day (up to 12 to 15 interviews), each lasting anywhere from 8 to 30 minutes, so be prepared for a lot of questioning. Depending on the program, interviews may be conducted by individual faculty members or by a panel consisting of three or more interviewers. Interviews are designed to measure applicants' interest in the specialty; to gauge the potential of each to contribute to the field; and to find out whether applicants would get along with other people in the department. Applicants are rarely pimped but will be expected to discuss any prior research or involvement in dermatology both intelligently and in detail.

For More Info . . .

- *American Academy of Dermatology Web site.* This site includes a mind-numbing description of accredited dermatology training programs along with a list of dermatology programs worldwide and of dermatology fellowships in North America. The information can be obtained by visiting:

    www.aad.org/professionals/residents/default.htm.

References

Rubenstein DS, Blauvelt A, Chen SC, Darling TN. The future of academic dermatology in the United States: report on the resident retreat for future physician-scientists, June 15–17, 2001. *J Am Acad Dermatol* 47(2):300–303, 2002.

Todd MM, Miller JJ, Ammirati CT. Dermatologic surgery training in residency. *Dermatol Surg* 28(7):547–549, 2002.

Emergency medicine (EM) has enjoyed considerable growth over the past few years, and with good reason. Relatively abundant free time, high pay (see Figure 4-3D), and the ability to integrate medicine with surgical procedures all add to this field's appeal. Fellowships are easily obtained for those who seek further training. Postresidency academic pursuits and fellowships can range from the exotic (international health, disaster/rescue medicine, and diving medicine) to the more commonplace (ultrasound, pediatrics, toxicology). EM is one of the only specialties in which a graduating resident may have a chance at an attending position straight out of residency, but these positions are becoming increasingly rare.

Over the past ten years, a number of hospitals and academic centers have added EM departments to their services, and many of these departments house residencies. Historically, EM is infamous for a high burnout rate. However, it is the youngest board-certified specialty (primary board status was not granted until 1989), so it is difficult to determine whether physicians who were recently trained in EM will show the same burnout rate in future years. It goes without saying that the ER can be stressful and that night shifts can drag on, but the EM resident's mantra is that he or she can always go home at the end of the day.

Residency programs in EM are unique in that they require either three or four years of total training. There has been much talk in the past about standardizing the amount of training required, but this has yet to materialize. In most cases, the internship year is integrated with the main EM training. For nonintegrated programs, a separate internship in medicine, surgery, or transitional medicine is required (although you do not have to do this at the same hospital). Obviously, this extra year can have a significant impact on an applicant's choice for training. If you are considering a three-year program, make sure that program offers the number of patients and level of acuity you'll need to acquire an adequate education in the three-year period.

The bulk of EM training time is spent in emergency rooms, learning resuscitation techniques, and treating both medical and trauma-related illnesses. However, residents also rotate through specialties such as medicine, pediatrics, OB/GYN, surgery, anesthesiology, and orthopedic surgery so that they can acquire a well-rounded knowledge and develop an eye for common emergencies in these fields. Different programs place "off-service" rotations in different years throughout the residency. Once you have interviewed at various programs, several factors will determine which programs you will rank more favorably. A recent study of residents just completing the EM match process within the last year or two revealed that the top five factors that they considered when choosing a program included friendliness (95%), environment (87%), perception of program during the interview day (81%), academics (76%), and location (74%).

Match Numbers

Competition for spots in EM residencies continues to intensify despite the addition of positions over the past several match years. In 1999 there were only 1063 total spots, while in 2005 that number had increased to 1332. In 2005, 1308 positions were filled, constituting a 98% fill rate (see Figures 4-3A and B). This high fill rate marks an upward trend in the number of applicants to

EMERGENCY MEDICINE

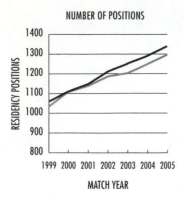

NUMBER OF POSITIONS

- POSITIONS OFFERED
- POSITIONS FILLED

A. Positions offered in emergency medicine and number filled.

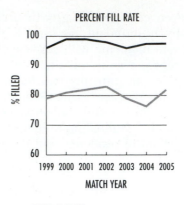

PERCENT FILL RATE

- TOTAL % FILLED
- U.S. % FILLED

B. Percentage of emergency medicine positions filled on Match Day.

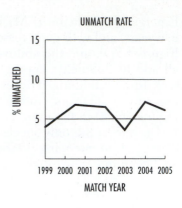

UNMATCH RATE

C. Percentage of U.S. seniors unmatched in emergency medicine on Match Day.

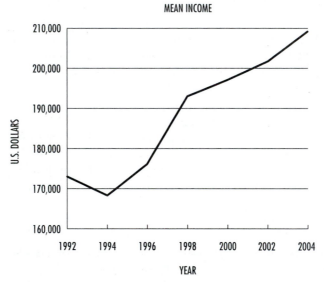

MEAN INCOME

D. Mean income of emergency medicine physicians in U.S. dollars.

FIGURES 4-3A–D

the field as EM residencies become increasingly competitive. In 2004, there were over 1500 applicants who ranked at least one EM program. In fact, 7% of all U.S. seniors who applied in EM in 2004 failed to match and had to scramble, representing an increase from previous years (see Figure 4-3C).

Application Tips

Given the competitive nature of EM, all aspects of the residency application are important. It is especially crucial to do well in an EM rotation and to ask for strong letters of recommendation from one of the attending physicians. (It would be even better to get a letter from the program director.) EM also remains a relatively close-knit field, especially at the attending level, so personal contact between attendings can be very helpful. If you have an attending who is willing to "go to bat for you," consider having him or her make a phone call to your top program closer to Match Day. (HINT: Don't make these calls all over; just focus on where you want to go.) Letters from surgery, medicine, pediatrics, or OB/GYN can also be well regarded, but your application must contain at least one very strong EM letter.

To improve your chances with a highly competitive program, consider doing an externship at that institution, especially if you are not particularly strong on paper—and be prepared to excel at that externship. Some competitive programs are known to use the USMLE Step 1 score to screen applications. Any research, especially in EM, should be highlighted, and the physician with whom you did the research should write the "nonclinical" letter for your application.

Your application should also reflect your outside interests. In EM perhaps more than in any other field, camaraderie is crucial during long shifts. People want to know that the resident with whom they are working is relatively fun and interesting. So let that show through in your application. All application and supporting material except for the dean's letter should be submitted by late September. Your dean's letter will be automatically added in early November, but some applicants will already be scheduling interviews at that point. The optimal number of applications to submit depends on the candidate's strength, but many suggest that 25 to 30 applications be submitted to yield 10 to 15 interviews. Timing of the interviews does not appear to affect selection committee rankings.

If you are very interested in a program but are not invited to interview, it is acceptable to call or e-mail that program and express your level of interest. Often, the program will review your application with your level of interest in mind to see if they can accommodate you, especially when interview spots open up later in the interview season.

Interview Tips

On your interview day, expect three to four interview sessions typically lasting 30 to 45 minutes each. Interviews are conducted by residency directors and other attendings. At some programs there may be a less formal interview with a resident, and at one or two of the larger county programs a charge nurse may conduct interviews as well. In general, EM interviewers are relaxed, friendly, and genuinely interested both in giving information about their programs and in learning more about the applicant's personality. It is important for EM interviewers to get a feel for the applicant's life outside of medicine.

As with other programs, it is also crucial for the applicant to determine specific factors that distinguish the program to which he or she is applying. So think about whether the program is county or private, three years or four, small or large, as all of these variables will have a considerable impact on your training. You should also come up with as many good, specific questions as you can regarding the hospital at which you are interviewing, as you will repeatedly be asked, "So do you have any questions?" Interviewers will also ask what other programs you are applying to. Answer politely and honestly, and do not "trash talk" other programs even if your interviewer does so. Be sure to write thank-you notes when you get home from the interview.

For More Info . . .

- *ACEP Student Information Packet.* This packet includes a directory of emergency medicine training programs. To obtain a copy, write or call:

  American College of Emergency Physicians
  P.O. Box 619911
  Dallas, TX 75261-9911
  (972) 550-0911
  (800) 798-1822
  www.acep.org

- Emergency Medicine Residents' Association (EMRA). In addition to the general information packet, you may wish to take out a student membership in EMRA. A $45 annual fee provides you with a subscription to *Annals of Emergency Medicine, ACEP News* (a monthly newsletter), *EM Resident* (a bimonthly newsletter), and access to specialty meetings and conferences. Since the medical student affiliate (MSA) branch of EMRA was created in 1992, most information has been geared toward residents. To enroll, call:

  Emergency Medicine Residents' Association
  (800) 798-1822
  www.emra.org

- Society for Academic Emergency Medicine (SAEM)
  901 North Washington Avenue
  Lansing, MI 48906-5137
  (517) 485-5484
  www.saem.org

- American Academy of Emergency Medicine (AAEM)
  611 East Wells Street
  Milwaukee, WI 53202
  (800) 884-2236
  www.aaem.org

- Delbridge TR. *Emergency Medicine in Focus: A Handbook for Medical Students and Prospective Residents.* A compact guide to the emergency medicine residency application process, it is available to EMRA/MSA members for $15. To order, call ACEP Publications, (800) 798-1822, ext. 6.

- Koscove EM. An applicant's evaluation of an emergency medicine internship and residency. *Ann Emerg Med* 19:774, 1990. This article offers an exhaustive collection of factors to consider when applying for and interviewing at EM training programs.

References

DeSantis M and Marco CA. Emergency medicine residency selection: factors influencing candidate decisions. *Acad Emerg Med* 12(6):559-561, 2005.

Gallagher EJ. Evolution of academic emergency medicine over a decade (1991–2001). *Acad Emerg Med* 9(10):995–1000, 2002.

Martin-Lee L, Park H, Overton DT. Does interview date affect match list position in the emergency medicine national residency matching program match? *Acad Emerg Med* 7(9):1022–1026, 2000.

Family practice (also called family medicine or family and community medicine) embraces the biopsychosocial model in its treatment of individuals and of the family as a whole. Students entering family practice have a strong commitment to primary care and enjoy the wide variety of patients and clinical problems encountered in this specialty, which spans medicine, pediatrics, OB/GYN, and surgery. This specialty has become significantly less popular with U.S. medical students over the past few years with the shift away from primary care, thus providing greater opportunities for international medical graduates (IMGs).

Family practice graduates enjoy good job prospects throughout the country. In one recent comprehensive study, 42.8% of 2723 family medicine physicians stated that they were very satisfied with their career. (This compares favorably to internal medicine, where 36.5% were very satisfied, and is similar to pediatrics, in which 48.1% were very satisfied.) In an academic center, the family practice graduate can often be an attending physician right out of residency. In some academic centers, the family physician is well respected for his or her breadth of knowledge and commitment to primary patient care. In other settings, the family physician may not be afforded due respect. Although subspecialty opportunities are limited, sports medicine, geriatrics, and adolescent medicine are growth areas. Geriatric medicine has a high career satisfaction rate, and opportunities in this area can only increase with the aging population. However, declining Medicare reimbursement rates may be an overriding negative for this specialty.

In family practice, there is relatively little consensus about the "best" programs to approach. You will generally be able to identify only the most "popular" programs, which depend on geographic region—university versus community versus rural. Note that curricula vary with geography, especially in the amount of obstetrics taught. The most formal training and education are afforded by a university setting; however, family practice may be negatively affected by strong internal medicine and specialty programs. Community-based programs that are the only residency in a particular hospital may offer some advantages. However, specialty training and didactic teaching often suffer.

Match Numbers

The percentage of U.S. graduates going into family medicine declined from 2000 to 2005, with 57% matched U.S. graduates in 2000 and 40% in 2005. The number of positions offered in family medicine also declined from 2000 to 2005 from 3206 to 2782 (13% decrease) (see Figures 4-4A–D).

Application Tips

Graduates with strong academic credentials will receive the red-carpet treatment in family medicine residency programs. This is especially true in academic medical centers, where good family medicine residents are valued as role models for students. Look for increased use of signing bonuses and other perks. Programs want to see a strong commitment to family medicine, and they particularly value a mature, well-rounded personality. Some programs may be sensitive to your reasons for choosing family practice over internal

FAMILY PRACTICE

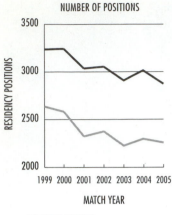

NUMBER OF POSITIONS

— POSITIONS OFFERED
— POSITIONS FILLED

A. Positions offered in family practice and number filled.

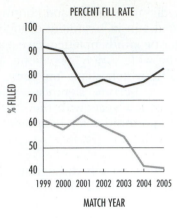

PERCENT FILL RATE

— TOTAL % FILLED
— U.S. % FILLED

B. Percentage of family practice positions filled on Match Day.

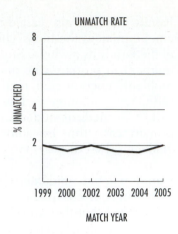

UNMATCH RATE

C. Percentage of U.S. seniors unmatched in family practice on Match Day.

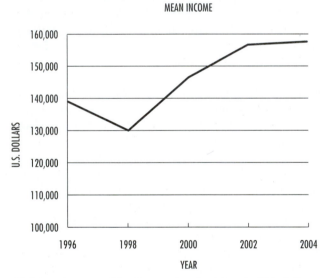

MEAN INCOME

D. Mean income of family practice physicians in U.S. dollars.

FIGURES 4-4A–D

medicine (especially primary care internal medicine) and will want to see a demonstrated interest in OB/GYN and pediatrics.

Interview Tips

Interviews are likely to be upbeat and supportive. Applicants have a particularly difficult task in information gathering, as assessment of the departments of pediatrics and OB/GYN is also important. The student needs to express the joy of patient care in and of itself whether or not a particular case is "interesting."

For More Info . . .

- American Academy of Family Physicians (AAFP)
  11400 Tomahawk Creek Parkway
  Leawood, KS 66211-2672
  (913) 906-6000
  (800) 274-2237
  www.aafp.org

- **AAFP student membership.** For a mere $10 per year, you will receive a subscription to the journal *American Family Physician*, which features practical articles on family medicine topics; the newsweekly *AAFP Reporter*; and a directory of family practice clerkships/preceptorships for students desiring clinical experience in family practice. Membership is limited to medical students at Liaison Committee on Medical Education (LCME)-accredited medical schools. To enroll, contact:

  > AAFP Membership Records
  > (800) 274-2237

- **AAFP publications.** The AAFP has a number of publications, many complimentary, aimed at medical students considering family practice. These include the following:
  - *Directory of Family Practice Residency Programs.* This is an annually revised database of family practice residencies that is considered more accurate, informative, and up-to-date than either FREIDA or the "Green Book." It is free to medical students through your school's family medicine department. Otherwise, the cost per copy is $10 for members and $15 for nonmembers.
  - *Reprint 300.* This booklet contains definitions of family practice and family physicians; it is free on request.
  - *Facts About Family Practice.* Geared toward number crunchers, this book includes detailed statistics about family practice. It costs $25 for members and $40 for nonmembers.
  - A *Medical Student's Guide to Strolling Through the Match.* This gives the what, when, where, why, and how of residency selection.
  - *Directory of Family Practice Clerkships/Preceptorships.*
  - *Residency Directory.* This gives information about more than 400 family practice residencies in the United States.
  - *Residency Information Packet.* A packet designed for medical students seeking statistical and informative data on family practice residency programs. Additional information enclosed includes a listing of all Accreditation Council for Graduate Medical Education (ACGME)-accredited family practice residency programs.

To order these publications, call the AAFP Order Department at (800) 274-2237.

References

Koehn NN, Fryer GE, Phillips RL, Miller JB, Green LA. The increase in international medical graduates in family medicine residency programs. *Fam Med* 34(6):429–435, 2002.

Leigh JP, Kravitz RL, Schembri M, Samuels SJ, Mobley S. Physician career satisfaction across specialties. *Arch Intern Med* 162:1577–1584, 2002.

Table 4-2. Internal Medicine Subspecialty Fellowships

Internal Medicine Subspecialty Fellowships
Cardiovascular disease
Clinical cardiac electrophysiology
Critical care medicine
Endocrinology, diabetes and metabolism
Gastroenterology
Geriatric medicine
Hematology
Hematology and oncology
Infectious disease
Interventional cardiology
Nephrology
Oncology
Pulmonary disease
Pulmonary disease and critical care medicine
Rheumatology
Sports medicine

A primary care medicine program does not rule out later subspecialty training.

Specialists enjoy a higher job satisfaction than generalists . . . at least for now.

Internal medicine programs are usually divided into categorical ("traditional") programs and primary care programs. Traditional medicine offers more of an inpatient focus plus electives for sampling different subspecialties. Residents in primary care medicine have more of an outpatient experience and often receive additional training in gynecology and pediatrics. However, this distinction is blurring as traditional programs increasingly require significant ambulatory care training.

Students are often attracted to internal medicine because it leaves the door open for further subspecialty training or generalist practice. On the other hand, students going into primary care internal medicine are often committed to primary care but are not as interested in the obstetrics, pediatrics, and surgical assisting experience offered by family practice. That said, many residents from traditional programs enter primary care, and conversely, many from primary care programs enter a subspecialty.

Although it has lost some popularity among U.S. graduates, internal medicine is still by far the most commonly chosen residency program. U.S. medical graduates filled 2659 residency positions in 2005 (up from 2590 in 2003). Many students are attracted to general internal medicine because of its emphasis on adult care, complex problem solving, and continuity of care. In many ways, too, internal medicine requires the skills that brought students to medical school in the first place: decision making, a vast knowledge base, and commitment to primary care. Students often seek the opportunity to provide in-depth and comprehensive care to adult patients without the need for frequent referral. In addition, many graduates now specifically gear their training toward a career as a hospitalist, including managing ICU patients.

More than half of those who choose internal medicine select one of 16 types of fellowships (see Table 4-2). Hence, there is enormous flexibility in internal medicine, with fields of interest including primary care ambulatory careers, highly technical specialties such as interventional cardiology, and purely hospital-based practices without ambulatory patients. A career in internal medicine is commonly combined with residencies in medicine-pediatrics, medicine-psychiatry, medicine-rehabilitation, medicine–preventive medicine, and medicine–emergency medicine.

In a recent career satisfaction survey conducted by Leigh et al., only 36.5% of internists described themselves as very satisfied with their field. Specialists were more satisfied. Specialties with the highest satisfaction rates, such as geriatrics (59.6% very satisfied), medical oncology (50.5% very satisfied), and infectious disease (50.0% very satisfied), actually ranked higher than orthopedic surgery, ophthalmology, and plastic surgery.

Match Numbers

Although the number of positions offered by internal medicine programs reached a record high of 4810 in 2000, only 93.4% of those positions were filled (see Figures 4-5A and B). Positions offered have decreased slightly, with 4662 having been offered in 2002, but are again on the rise, with 4768 positions offered in 2005. Fill rates have increased from the steady rate of 94% (1998–2002) to 97% in 2004 and 2005. Only 55% of positions were filled by

INTERNAL MEDICINE

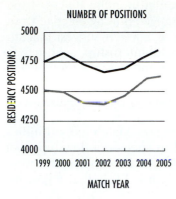

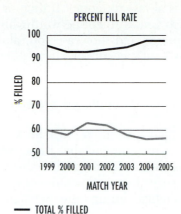

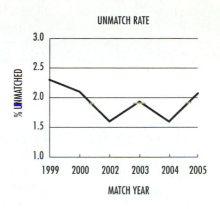

A. Positions offered in internal medicine and number filled.

B. Percentage of internal medicine positions filled on Match Day.

C. Percentage of U.S. seniors unmatched in internal medicine on Match Day.

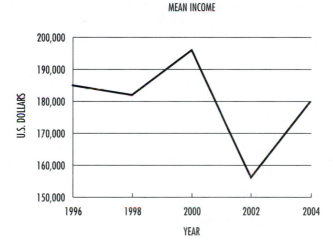

D. Mean income of internists in U.S. dollars.

FIGURES 4-5A–D

U.S. medical graduates from 2003 to 2005, so the field continues to offer great opportunities to IMGs. Some fellowships have become competitive, particularly cardiology and gastroenterology.

Application Tips

U.S. graduates do not have a difficult time matching into one of the numerous excellent programs available. At the same time, there is considerable variability among program directors and committees with regard to which part of the application is weighted most heavily. Very competitive programs value high grades in medical clerkships and subinternships as well as high class rank. Interest or accomplishments in research are highly regarded in academic programs. Internal medicine residents must also be good teachers of medical students if they are to make medicine clerkships work well, so an interest in teaching is always welcome! If there is a particular program that is of special interest to you, it might be worthwhile to arrange an away elective to solidify your interest and showcase your ability. Many advisers suggest that students opt for a subspecialty elective rather than a subinternship, as it may be easier to make a good impression in a less rigorous and perhaps more academic subspecialty experience. It is reasonable to apply to at least ten programs. Do not rank a program unless you want to train there.

In internal medicine, there will be some good post-Match opportunities. Some advisers recommend that those interested in specific fellowships look for programs that have such fellowships available, particularly in the more competitive specialties (e.g., cardiology). However, it is likely that fellowship choices will change during residency training.

Interview Tips

There are no typical schedules or interview days in internal medicine. Several interviews lasting 15 to 30 minutes each are probably the rule. Often, time is spent giving applicants information about the strengths of the particular program. It is very rare for applicants to present cases or be asked factual questions. However, program directors will almost always want to know about your choice of primary care versus various specialties. There is no "right answer" to these questions. Those going into primary care might be seen in a positive light as future general internal medicine faculty. By the same token, those going into specialty training might fill important fellowship slots and are more likely to participate in research. In any case, be prepared to address your career interests, discuss why you are interested in a particular program, and in a non-egocentric fashion, talk about what your personal strong points may be. An excellent work ethic is a quality that all program directors will value.

For More Info . . .

- American College of Physicians (ACP)
190 North Independence Mall West
Philadelphia, PA 19106-1572
(800) 523-1546, ext. 2600
(215) 351-2600
www.acponline.org

- American College of Preventive Medicine (ACPM)
1307 New York Avenue, N.W., Suite 200
Washington, D.C. 20005
(202) 466-2044
www.acpm.org

- American Geriatrics Society (AGS)
Empire State Building
350 Fifth Avenue, Suite 801
New York, NY 10118
(212) 308-1414
www.americangeriatrics.org

48

■ American Gastroenterological Association
4930 Del Ray Avenue
Bethesda, MD 20814
(301) 654-2055
www.gastro.org

Reference

Leigh JP, Kravitz RL, Schembri M, Samuels SJ, Mobley S. Physician career satisfaction across specialties. *Arch Intern Med* 162:1577–1584, 2002.

MED-PEDS

Internal medicine-pediatrics (med-peds) is a growing field in medicine. This combined program began in 1967 (even before the first family medicine residency) and currently has more than 4500 practitioners nationwide and 1500 residents. Similar to family medicine training, med-peds attracts students interested in working closely with both children and adults. In addition, this field is sought by those who find continuity of care and close, long-term doctor-patient relationships rewarding.

The four-year med-peds residency, unlike family medicine residency, does not include any formal obstetrical or surgical training and instead provides more thorough training in adult and pediatric medicine. Once the four-year residency is complete, med-peds physicians are board eligible in both internal medicine and pediatrics. On average, board passing rates are greater than or equal to categorical internal medicine or pediatric physicians.

Med-peds graduates have the ability to fill unique niches in the health care community. They care for children, adolescents, adults, and especially adults with chronic "pediatric" health conditions (e.g., congenital heart disease, cystic fibrosis, etc.). Currently, approximately 78% of med-peds practitioners work in a primary care practice while 22% have subspecialized in one of more than 24 subspecialty fellowships open to med-peds physicians.

Match Numbers

Currently, there are approximately 105 med-peds programs offering around 400 first-year positions, accounting for 10% of internal medicine and 15% of pediatric residency positions nationwide. In general, the limited number of med-peds positions nationally makes med-peds programs more competitive than their parent categorical programs. Even so, most determined applicants do not have a problem obtaining a position. In 2005, 87.2% of the 390 offered positions were filled and, of those, 70.5% were filled with U.S. seniors (see Figures 4-6A–D).

Please note that no surveys have been done to calculate the mean income for med-peds physicians, but it is estimated to be similar to that of other generalists (peds, IM, family practice).

MED-PEDS

NUMBER OF POSITIONS

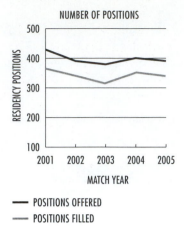

PERCENT FILL RATE

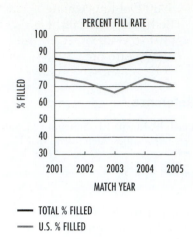

A. Positions offered in med-peds and numbers filled.

B. Percentage of med-peds positions filled on Match Day.

FIGURES 4-6A–B

Application Tips

Matching in med-peds is more competitive than categorical pediatrics or medicine, so students should apply to 15 to 20 programs and hope for a comfortable ten interviews. Programs will want to sense your desire to work with children and adults. Extracurricular activities and your personal statement are perfect places in which to emphasize this desire. In addition, strong grades in both pediatric and internal medicine clerkships as well as excellent letters of support from faculty members in both fields are essential. Finding the time to successfully complete a subinternship in internal medicine, pediatrics, or both may help your application.

Interview Tips

During the interview process, you will interview with both the internal medicine and pediatrics department at each institution, which usually makes the interview a two-day event. Programs will want to see well-rounded, dedicated candidates with a strong desire to work with both children and adults. Candidates should be able to confidently explain why they chose to pursue med-peds training instead of family practice. In addition, as with all generalist fields in medicine, excellent communication skills are highly favored. Make sure you schedule enough time between interviews to keep yourself refreshed. The two-day interviews can be tiring, and you want to be your best on each day.

For More Info . . .

- National Med-Peds Residents' Association (NMPRA) (www.medpeds.org)
- Internal Medicine and Pediatrics 101 (www.aap.ort/sections/med-peds/101.htm)

- Caring for Adults—A Comparison of Three Residency Options (Family Medicine, Internal Medicine, and Internal Medicine and Pediatrics) (www.medpeds.org/pdf/three.pdf)
- The Medical Student Guide to the Combined Internal Medicine and Pediatrics Residency Training (www.medpeds.org/PDF/StudentGuide.pdf)
- Guidelines for Combined Internal Medicine/Pediatrics Residency Training (www.acgme.org/acWebsite/RRC_sharedDocs/sh_medPedREq.pdf)
- American Academy of Pediatrics (AAP) Med-Peds Section (www.aap.org/sections/med-peds/)

Reference

Frohna JG, Melgar T, Mueller C, Boder S. Internal medicine-pediatrics residency training: current program trends and outcomes. *Acad Med* 79(6): June 2004.

NEUROLOGY

Neurology has greatly benefited from the recent explosion in technological research. Over the past few years, the specialty has grown and changed direction to the point at which it is now geared more toward treatment, traditionally its least emphasized area. Most neurology physicians and residents feel that primary care physicians can take increasing responsibility for such chronic problems as stroke, headaches, and uncomplicated seizures. However, more complex neurological problems will still require the care of a specialist, and management of acute stroke is now more sophisticated, with a high demand for graduates to help in the emergency room setting. Job opportunities for neurologists seeking private practices are thus readily available at present. In fact, some studies project a critical shortage (up to 30%) in the supply of neurologists by the year 2010.

Neurology requires a three-year residency program preceded by an internship year in medicine, surgery, or transitional medicine. It generally works in the resident's favor to choose a medicine preliminary program, as such programs tend to be more relevant to later training in neurology. Look for preliminary program opportunities that might provide the flexibility to do neurosurgery electives, ophthalmology, or even neuroanatomy. Also keep in mind that the patient population may influence the quality and focus of training in certain areas (e.g., trauma-related neurologic diseases, HIV disease, or such chronic problems as stroke and dementia). A few schools have combined psychiatry and neurology training in one department.

Match Numbers

The number of positions offered by neurology programs increased from 541 in 2002 to 558 in 2004 (see Figure 4-7A). In 2006, the unmatch rate for U.S. seniors jumped from 4% to 7% (see Figure 4-7C). Overall, applicants applied to 20 programs and had an average of 5.5 interviews. Most unmatched applicants have been IMGs. The neurology Match is at present a "two-tier" system for PGY-2 positions in that PGY-2 positions that did not fill in the previous Match are offered alongside the PGY-2 positions scheduled to begin in a year and a half. The number of vacancies left after the first-tier Match has dropped from 111 in 1996 to 38 in the 2006 Match—a clear sign of improving conditions for the neurology Match.

NEUROLOGY

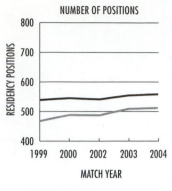

A. Positions offered in neurology and number filled.

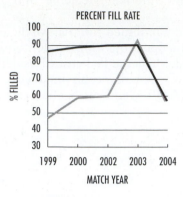

B. Percentage of neurology positions filled on Match Day.

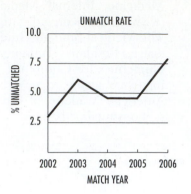

C. Percentage of U.S. seniors unmatched in neurology on Match Day.

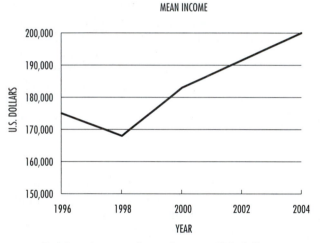

D. Mean income of neurologists in U.S. dollars.

FIGURES 4-7A–D

Application Tips

Positions for neurology residencies are filled through an early match, so applicants must be diligent in completing their applications as soon as possible. Deadlines for most programs are in November or December; all information should be submitted by October. Senior neurology rotations should be completed in the summer before the fourth year to ensure early letters of recommendation. This is one field in which the reputation of the letter writer counts as much as the letter's substance. Generally, you should ask for a letter from the best-known and most senior members of the neurology faculty, since their voices will resonate the loudest with the review committee. On another note, away rotations at institutions of interest could help, although opinion is divided on this issue.

To strengthen your application, you should include tangible proof of your commitment to the field of neurology, such as research experience, clinical volunteer experience, and publications. Some programs will also look at the location of your internship institution and the type of internship to which you applied. In general, many programs prefer a medical internship located at either the same institution or a similarly prestigious one.

Interview Tips

Interviews range from individual sessions lasting about 30 to 45 minutes to group sessions conducted by a panel of faculty members. Each program has a different style, so be sure to ask about their format when you call to schedule the appointment. Most of the time, the questions will be designed to gauge your dedication to the field. In addition to the common interview fare (see Chapter 11), some interviewers will ask applicants to describe their research projects or to offer their opinions on ethical issues in neurologic diagnosis and treatment. Some neurology programs have weaknesses in more recent specialty areas such as neuro-oncology, neurogenetics, and neuro-immunology. It is thus important to determine the department's preparedness to teach these areas.

For More Info . . .

- A student information packet can be obtained by calling or writing:

  American Academy of Neurology (AAN)
  1080 Montreal Avenue
  St. Paul, MN 55116
  (800) 879-1960
  (651) 695-2717
  www.aan.com

- Other sources of information include:

  American Board of Psychiatry and Neurology (ABPN)
  500 Lake Cook Road, Suite 335
  Deerfield, IL 60015-5249
  (847) 945-7900
  www.abpn.com

  San Francisco Match Neurology Matching Program
  P.O. Box 7584
  San Francisco, CA 94120-7584
  (415) 447-0350
  Fax: (415) 561-8535
  E-mail: help@sfmatch.org
  www.sfmatch.org

References

Corboy JR, Boudreau E, Morgenlander JC, Rudnicki S, Coyle PK. Neurology residency training at the millennium. *Neurology* 58:1454–1460, 2002.
Ringel SP, Vickrey BG, Keran CM, Bieber J, Bradley WG. Training the future neurology workforce. *Neurology* 54(2):480–484, 2002.

Neurological surgery is an extremely rewarding surgical specialty, providing opportunities to participate in the most critical of clinical situations, undertake advanced clinical or basic research, and become involved in an ever-changing and challenging field. However, this specialty is notorious for remaining one of the most competitive fields in medicine despite its demanding schedules and high attrition rate.

Neurosurgery requires a lifestyle choice as well as a professional one.

Neurosurgeons provide operative and nonoperative management of lesions of the brain, spinal cord, and peripheral nerves and their supporting structures. Neurosurgeons also participate in the critical care and rehabilitation of brain and spinal cord trauma as well as other neurologic disorders, including chronic pain, Parkinson's, and epilepsy. With advances in imaging technologies, gene transfer therapy, and tissue implantation, the field of neurosurgery will continue to be an extremely exciting specialty for many years to come.

Specialty training in neurological surgery begins with a 12-month internship in general surgery followed by six years of residency in neurosurgery. Neurosurgical ICU and floor management usually begins during the second year of residency. A minimum of 36 months of training must be spent in clinical neurosurgery along with three months in clinical neurology and three months in neuroradiology. Depending on the program, operative experience and patient responsibility usually increase every year, culminating during your last year of neurosurgical residency. Within your neurosurgical experience, residents are usually required to participate in at least one full year of research, either basic or clinical. Many different hospital environments are typically involved in residency training, including county, private, and VA facilities. Upon completion of a neurological surgery residency, residents should be proficient in operative procedures involving tumors, complex spine, pediatrics, and vascular neurosurgery; should efficiently and effectively manage the clinical care of neurosurgical patients; and should be able to critically evaluate relevant neurosurgical research. Some programs offer fellowship training within or after the completion of a residency program or offer training experiences at other campuses and institutions both in the United States and abroad.

Match Numbers

Despite a recent drop in the number of applicants in the field since 1995, the number of registration and rank-order list (ROL) submissions has leveled off over the past several years. In 2004 and 2005, 282 and 257 applicants submitted ROLs, respectively. Of the 257 applicants who submitted ROLs in January 2005, 222 were ranked and 154 matched, leaving only two positions unfilled (see Figure 4-8A). Of those who applied to neurological surgery programs, 85% of U.S. seniors matched (see Figure 4-8C), whereas only 25% of IMGs matched. The average USMLE Step 1 score for applicants who matched in January 2004 and 2005 was 235.

Application Tips

Positions in neurological surgery are offered through the San Francisco Match Neurosurgery Matching Program (www.sfmatch.org). Given that neurological surgery is intensely competitive, applicants are expected to demonstrate a

NEUROSURGERY

NUMBER OF POSITIONS

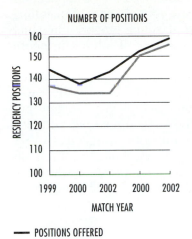

PERCENT FILL RATE

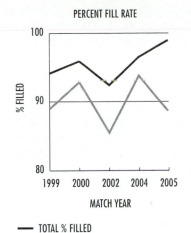

UNMATCH RATE

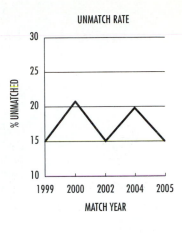

— POSITIONS OFFERED
— POSITIONS FILLED

— TOTAL % FILLED
— U.S. % FILLED

A. Positions offered in neurosurgery and number filled.

B. Percentage of neurosurgery positions filled on Match Day.

C. Percentage of U.S. seniors unmatched in neurosurgery on Match Day.

FIGURES 4-8A–C

number of accomplishments prior to application, such as a high USMLE Step 1 score (higher than the 80th percentile), election to AΩA, a postgraduate degree, or honors in clinical rotations (e.g., general surgery). Yet while any or all accolades will complement an application, there are other ways to improve your chances for interviews. Given that neurological surgery is an early Match specialty, the earlier your application is completed and submitted, the better your chance for an interview. Another strategy to improve your chances is to participate in a clinical externship at your institution of interest, especially if your home institution does not have a neurological surgery division or department of its own. Most institutions require proof of good standing at your medical school, complete immunization records, health and medical coverage, and various other personal information months prior to the start of an externship. So apply early, and vigorously follow up with these institutions to ensure your externship position.

One goal of completing an externship is to obtain letters of recommendation from neurosurgeons in that program, including but not limited to the chairman and/or the residency program director. Many programs look favorably on letters of recommendation from neurosurgeons, especially if they are from well-known institutions. If it is not possible to complete an externship at another institution, you should at least participate in a neurological surgery elective or a subinternship in general surgery with an emphasis on neurosurgery. Experiences in academic neurological surgery are always beneficial. Finally, participating in research at your medical institution is always a good tactic and bodes well for your application, especially if that research involves topics closely related to neurological surgery.

All application and supporting materials for the Match should be submitted by late August. The average applicant submits 38 applications and interviews at 10 to 11 programs. The optimal number of applications depends on your strength as a candidate, but it is recommended that you submit 30 to 40 applications and go to as many interviews as possible to increase your chances of matching. There are many factors to consider when you are selecting programs in which to apply, including program strength, location, and type of interest in neurosurgery (not every program is equally strong in all areas of neurological surgery). One strategy for deciding which programs to approach is to ask neurological surgery residents at your home institution or at other institutions with a neurological surgery department about different neurological surgery programs. Yet another strategy is to attend one of the large annual neurosurgical meetings—e.g., the American Association of Neurological Surgeons (AANS) or the Congress of Neurological Surgeons (CNS). These strategies can significantly bolster your knowledge of what to look for in a program while also strengthening your ability to distinguish the different kinds and structures of neurological surgery programs.

Interview Tips

Most interviews last a single day with a dinner either the night before or immediately following the interview day. Some programs reserve more than one day for interviews, but this is usually the case only in the larger programs. Most visits consist of similar activities, including grand rounds, campus/hospital tours, interviews, and meetings with residents. Individual interviews typically last 15 to 30 minutes. It is often helpful to read about programs before interviewing, as most interviewers will ask if you have any questions about their program. Frequent topics of interest include available research opportunities, the number and variety of cases seen per year, and the amount of operative experience gained. Finally, it is always handy to have a photograph, a CV, and reprints of your publications with you during your interview.

For More Info...

- American Association of Neurological Surgeons
  5550 Meadowbrook Drive
  Rolling Meadows, IL 60008
  (847) 378-0500
  (888) 566-AANS
  www.aans.org

- Congress of Neurological Surgeons
  www.neurosurgery.org/cns/index.asp

- American Board of Neurological Surgery (ABNS)
  6550 Fannin Street, Suite 2139
  Houston, TX 77030
  (713) 441-6015
  www.abns.org

- San Francisco Match Neurosurgery Matching Program
  P.O. Box 7584
  San Francisco, CA 94120-7584
  (415) 447-0350
  Fax: (415) 561-8535
  E-mail: help@sfmatch.org
  www.sfmatch.org

OB/GYN is a field that is limited only by the type of patients treated: female. From gynecologic evaluation to total obstetrical care, the obstetrician/gynecologist is essential to providing a continuum of women's health care. In addition, about half of all women utilize the obstetrician/gynecologist as their sole source of health care. Therefore, the obstetrician/gynecologist is in the unique position of providing both medical and surgical care.

OB/GYN has benefited from impressive biomedical advances in recent years; enhanced maternal care and high-risk pregnancy management, in vitro fertilization, and increasing numbers of laparoscopic-assisted and in utero surgeries have lured candidates to the field. For the individual who appreciates interacting with patients in an outpatient setting but also enjoys high-tech procedural and surgical opportunities, OB/GYN may be the right choice. There are, however, some issues that make OB/GYN more problematic. The high cost of malpractice coverage and the threat of litigation, for example, have become national issues. Residency program directors are aware of these concerns, and the vast majority of programs are incorporating some degree of formal medical-legal education into their residency curricula. Added to this has been the increasing competition that has resulted from the advanced training of nurse practitioners and nurse midwives to perform obstetrical services.

The length of residency training in OB/GYN is four years. The initial two years of training concentrate on obtaining competencies in general obstetrics, routine gynecology, outpatient care, gynecologic oncology, and basic surgical skills. The final two years involve increasing exposure to specialty areas. The upper-level resident must continuously hone teaching, management, and leadership skills. After finishing residency, a candidate must complete two years of practice before becoming board eligible. Further specialization in gynecologic oncology, maternal-fetal medicine, urogynecology, or reproductive endocrinology requires an additional two to three years of training.

When evaluating potential residency programs, candidates should make certain that a wide range of training opportunities will be available. Candidates should keep in mind, for example, that hospital programs with religious affiliations may offer little or no experience in many aspects of fertility management, in vitro fertilization, and therapeutic and elective abortion.

Match Numbers

OB/GYN residencies remain somewhat competitive. Although fewer deliveries are being performed by OB/GYN physicians, the number of residency positions has remained stable at 1144 (compared to 1142 in 2004). In 2005, 1083 of 1144 positions (94.7%) were filled in the Match. Although the total percentage of positions filled has remained relatively stable over the past several years, the percentage filled by U.S. graduates has dropped from around 80% in 2002 to around 70% in 2004 and 2005 (see Figures 4-9A and 4-9B). At the same time, the number of spots filled by IMGs has risen steadily over the past five years, with around 30% filled by IMGs in 2004 and 2005 (see Figure 4-9B). Residents work long hours and are often sleep deprived. Most welcome limits on their work schedule. Partly as a result of high levels of concern about

OB/GYN has an exciting mix of clinic work and operating-room time.

Malpractice insurance cost in OB/GYN is becoming a national issue.

YOUR SPECIALTY AND THE MATCH

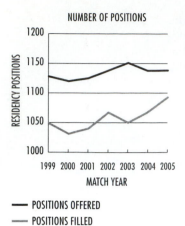

NUMBER OF POSITIONS

— POSITIONS OFFERED
— POSITIONS FILLED

A. Positions offered in obstetrics and gynecology and number filled.

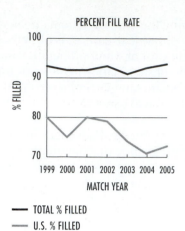

PERCENT FILL RATE

— TOTAL % FILLED
— U.S. % FILLED

B. Percentage of obstetrics and gynecology positions filled on Match Day.

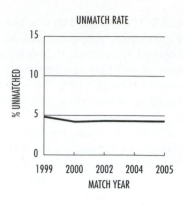

UNMATCH RATE

C. Percentage of U.S. seniors unmatched in obstetrics and gynecology on Match Day.

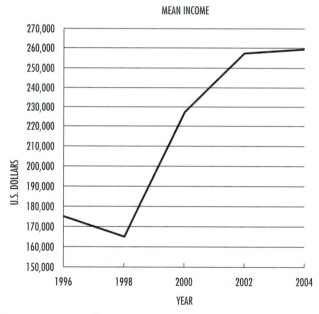

MEAN INCOME

D. Mean income of obstetricians and gynecologists in U.S. dollars.

FIGURES 4-9A–D

malpractice, career satisfaction is relatively low, with only 34.4% of practitioners reporting that they are very satisfied with the field. Those practicing only gynecology also report low job satisfaction, with only 27.3% reporting that they are very satisfied with their specialty.

Application Tips

In 1992, a survey of OB/GYN residency program directors evaluated the most important aspects of the application. Grades, deans' letters, and USMLE scores were rated as the most important criteria influencing the likelihood of obtaining an interview. The interview itself was also considered to be key. Resident program directors in OB/GYN know that USMLE scores predict success on board pass rates. Some prestigious programs have further suggested that students try to complete away rotations at institutions that interest them, as a good impression on an away rotation improves the chances of being offered an interview. Strong evaluations in surgical rotations will similarly increase the applicant's strength. All application materials should be submitted as early as possible, usually by October.

Interview Tips

OB/GYN interviews are usually conducted in December and January. When you call to schedule, be aware that many programs have only a limited time period within which to interview large groups of applicants. So the earlier you submit your application, the more choices you'll have. Interview schedules may run long, lasting from 8 a.m. to 5 p.m., and generally consist of three to four interviews of 30 to 45 minutes each. Interviews may be individual or group depending on the program. When you interview, you should bear in mind that the "miracle of birth" is not a good enough reason for your having chosen this specialty. Remember, OB/GYN programs want to attract applicants who will become competent surgeons but also have the capability to provide good primary care for women. So be prepared to present a case, discuss ethical issues related to the specialty, and explain why you want to be an obstetrician/gynecologist. If you've done basic or clinical research, know your work inside out, for you will be questioned on it. Highly rated applicants are seen as future competent surgeons as well as excellent potential primary care physicians for women. Applicants should be well versed in all important aspects of women's health. For the most part, interviews are cordial and informal, offering the interviewer an opportunity to assess your personality.

For More Info . . .

- Student information packets are available by calling or writing:

  American College of Obstetricians and Gynecologists (ACOG)
  409 12th Street, S.W.
  P.O. Box 96920
  Washington, D.C. 20090-6920
  (202) 638-5577
  www.acog.org

References

Bell JG, Kanellitsas I, Shaffer L. Selection of obstetrics and gynecology residents on the basis of medical school performance. *Am J Obstet Gynecol* 186(5):1091–1094, 2002.

Defoe DM, Power ML, Holzman GB, Carpentieri A, Schulkin J. Long hours and little sleep: work schedules of residents in obstetrics and gynecology. *Obstet Gynecol* 97(6):1015–1018, 2001.

Leigh JP, Kravitz RL, Schembri M, Samuels SJ, Mobley S. Physician career satisfaction across specialties. *Arch Intern Med* 162:1577–1584, 2002.

Metheny WP, Ling FW, Holzman GB, Mitchum MJ. Answers to applicant selection from a directory of residency programs in obstetrics and gynecology. *Obstet Gynecol* 88(1):133–136, 1996.

Moreno-Hunt C, Gilbert WM. Current status of obstetrics and gynecology resident medical-legal education: a survey of program directors. *Obstet Gynecol* 106(6):1382-1384, 2005.

Taylor CA, Weinstein L, Mayhew HE. The process of resident selection: a view from the residency director's desk. *Obstet Gynecol* 85(2):299–303, 1995.

OPHTHALMOLOGY

Understand the differences between ophthalmology and optometry, and their political turf battles.

Thanks in large part to innovations in surgical and laser techniques, ophthalmology has recently taken off as a high-tech surgical and medical specialty. Although optometrists have taken over some of the functions that were previously the domain of the ophthalmologist, new procedures and technologies have made the field even more attractive to medical students. Since the work is mostly outpatient with little night call, the field has particular appeal even in comparison to other surgical specialties—although the relative competitiveness of surgical subspecialty positions is difficult to determine and changes over time. Perhaps surprisingly, a recent survey reports relatively low career satisfaction among ophthalmologists, with 41.4% expressing a high level of satisfaction—a level falling below general surgery, orthopedic surgery, and urology.

Residencies in ophthalmology require one year of internship followed by three years of specialty training. Residents often rotate through both surgical and nonsurgical rotations, learning surgical techniques as well as the medical diagnosis and management of eye diseases. Board eligibility is achieved immediately after the completion of residency. Currently, there is no certification for subspecialties. However, residents can tailor their training to reflect areas of interest such as cataract, glaucoma, or retinal surgery. Fellowship opportunities following residency training in ophthalmology include cataract/general, cornea, glaucoma, LASIK/refractive, neuro, ocular pathology, oculoplastics, pediatric, and vitreo-retinal.

Match Numbers

Ophthalmology remains one of the most competitive specialties. In 2002, there were 440 positions offered and 438 positions filled, and in 2004 and 2005 the numbers remained similar (see Figure 4-10A). Evidence of the highly competitive nature of this field includes the number of applications per applicant (43), the average USMLE score for successful applicants (229), and the low number of unfilled positions over the past several years (two to seven). The nonmatch rate for U.S. seniors has declined over the past few years from around 22% in 2002 to 14% in 2005, but this percentage continues to remain high when compared to other specialties (see Figure 4-10C). IMGs continue to fare poorly, with a nonmatch rate of around 75%.

Application Tips

Positions in ophthalmology residencies are offered primarily through the Ophthalmology Matching Program run by the San Francisco Match. Applications should be submitted by late August and ROLs by January. Match results are announced in time for applicants to learn their results before the deadline for the PGY-1 preliminary program sponsored by the National Resident Matching Program (NRMP). Given the competition to enter the field, the potential applicant should concentrate on doing well on the

OPHTHALMOLOGY

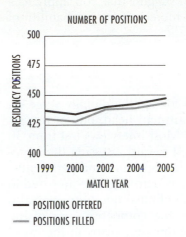

A. Positions offered in ophthalmology and number filled.

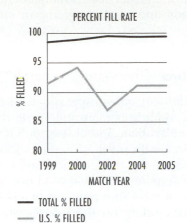

B. Percentage of ophthalmology positions filled on Match Day.

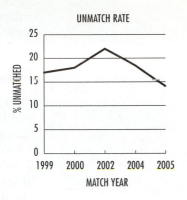

C. Percentage of U.S. seniors unmatched in ophthalmology on Match Day.

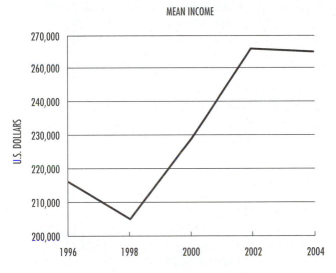

D. Mean income of ophthalmologists in U.S. dollars.

FIGURES 4-10A–D

USMLE Step 1, in core senior electives, and in the senior ophthalmology rotation. Some programs use election to AΩA as a screening tool! Applicants try to push the number of audition electives to the maximum allowed by the medical school—usually two or three. Supportive evaluations and recommendations from the senior ophthalmology faculty will clinch a strong application.

Since this is another field in which most department heads know one another, connections can play an important part in getting you that interview. In addition, any research experience, especially work resulting in publications and/or presentations, should be included in your CV. At present, most applicants are advised to submit about 20 to 35 applications in the hope of getting ten or so interviews. Many advisers also suggest that you apply to a mix of strong and weak programs in order to increase your probability of matching.

Interview Tips

As with other surgical subspecialties, interviews for ophthalmology verge on the formal. Applicants often meet with the department head, one or two senior faculty members, and at least one resident. Most interviews last from 30 to 45 minutes, with many of the questions geared toward assessing the applicant's interest in the field, clinical and research background, and personality. If you have done research that you hope will give you an edge, be prepared to discuss your project in a polished manner. Some clinical questions may also be asked, depending on the interviewer. Given the competitiveness of the field, interviewers sometimes ask about your contingency plans in the event that you don't match in ophthalmology.

For More Info . . .

- *Envision Ophthalmology: A Practical Guide to Ophthalmology as a Career Choice.* A free publication of the American Academy of Ophthalmology (AAO), this booklet includes general information about the application process as well as a practical discussion of factors to consider in selecting and assessing an ophthalmology program. To receive this excellent career guide, call or write:

  > American Academy of Ophthalmology
  > P.O. Box 7424
  > San Francisco, CA 94120-7424
  > (415) 561-8500
  > www.aao.org

- Further information can be obtained from the following organizations:

  > American Board of Ophthalmology (ABO)
  > 111 Presidential Boulevard, Suite 241
  > Bala Cynwyd, PA 19004-1075
  > (610) 664-1175
  > www.abop.org

  > Glaucoma Research Foundation (to inquire about research opportunities)
  > 490 Post Street, Suite 1427
  > San Francisco, CA 94102
  > (415) 986-3162
  > (800) 826-6693
  > www.glaucoma.org

  > San Francisco Match Ophthalmology Matching Program
  > P.O. Box 7584
  > San Francisco, CA 94120-7584
  > (415) 447-0350
  > Fax: (415) 561-8535
  > E-mail: help@sfmatch.org
  > www.sfmatch.org

References

Andriole DA, Schechtman KB, Ryan K, Whelan A, Diemer K. How competitive is my surgical specialty? *Am J Surg* 84(1):1–5, 2002.

Leigh JP, Kravitz RL, Schembri M, Samuels SJ, Mobley S. Physician career satisfaction across specialties. *Arch Intern Med* 162(14):1577-1584, 2002.

ORTHOPEDICS

Orthopedic surgery continues to be a rewarding field. Specialists have the opportunity to combine surgical techniques and orthopedic hardware (e.g., microsurgery and joint prostheses) with work in physical rehabilitation for the treatment of acute and chronic orthopedic problems. In addition, earnings for orthopedic surgeons continue to be well above average (see Figure 4-11D). However, increasing professional liability insurance premiums and overhead costs are reducing overall compensation. On the whole, 47.1% of orthopedic surgeons evaluate their career as very satisfactory, which represents a relatively high percentage among medical specialties.

Residencies require at least five years of training, with up to two years spent in general surgery or other approved medical or surgical residencies and the last three years spent in an orthopedic surgery program. A post-residency practice period is required before you become board eligible. Subspecialty training is available in hand surgery, spinal surgery, sports medicine, orthopedic trauma, and pediatric orthopedics.

Match Numbers

In 2005, 605 of 610 positions were filled in the Match, making orthopedic surgery among the most competitive surgical specialties. The number of positions offered by orthopedic surgery programs increased from 589 in 2004 to 610 in 2005 (see Figure 4-11A). The vast majority of positions continue to be filled by U.S. medical graduates, with only 35 to 45 IMGs per year matching in orthopedic programs over the past several years (see Figure 4-11B). The unmatched rate for U.S. seniors continues to remain around 15% (see Figure 4-11C).

Application Tips

Bernstein et al. recently summarized the process and criteria that orthopedic surgery residency program directors have used for selection of residents. Academic credentials, including class rank and USMLE scores, are heavily relied on. The prestige of AΩA election is now widely recognized as well; 54% of all successful candidates are members of AΩA. Also well established and documented in the Bernstein study is the enormous importance of performing the audition elective, or "orthopedic clerkship," at the program director's institution.

The interview process in orthopedics is directed toward "getting to know" the applicant and is probably not useful in distinguishing one outstanding applicant from another. However, 5% of programs tested manual skills and 18% used clinical scenarios as part of the interview process. While the assumption is often made that research is a necessity to match in orthopedics, this is not supported by the literature. Also important to note is a recent study by Dale et

One in seven U.S. seniors went unmatched in orthopedic surgery.

ORTHOPEDICS

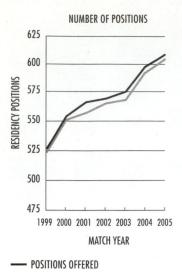

NUMBER OF POSITIONS

— POSITIONS OFFERED
— POSITIONS FILLED

A. Positions offered in orthopedics and number filled.

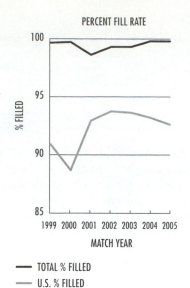

PERCENT FILL RATE

— TOTAL % FILLED
— U.S. % FILLED

B. Percentage of orthopedic positions filled on Match Day.

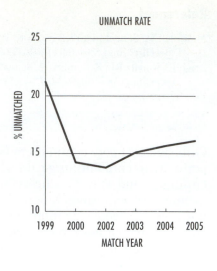

UNMATCH RATE

C. Percentage of U.S. seniors un-matched in orthopedics on Match Day.

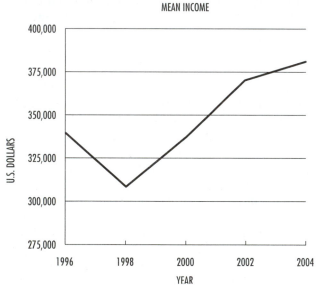

MEAN INCOME

D. Mean income of orthopedic surgeons in U.S. dollars.

FIGURES 4-11A–D

High board scores, AΩA, many honors, and research are the keys to success.

al., which found that many candidates "falsified research citations on their applications to orthopedic programs."

Interview Tips

Interviews in orthopedic surgery are extremely difficult to obtain, so if you are offered one, it means that you've proven yourself academically. As stated, the Bernstein review suggests that 18% of program directors do use clinical scenarios, so be prepared, at a minimum, to present an interesting or memorable case. If you have done research, be particularly careful to accurately describe your findings and their significance. Interviews are usually conducted from mid-November to early February.

For More Info . . .

- For a brochure on careers in orthopedic surgery, call or write:

     American Academy of Orthopaedic Surgeons (AAOS)
     6300 North River Road
     Rosemont, IL 60018-4262
     (847) 823-7186
     (800) 346-AAOS
     www.aaos.org

References

Bernstein AD, Jazrawi LM, DellaValle CJ, Zuckerman JD. Orthopedic resident selection criteria. *J Bone Joint Surg Am* 84:2090–2096, 2002.
Dale JA, Schmitt CM, Crosby LA. Misrepresentation of research criteria by orthopedic residency applicants. *J Bone Joint Surg Am* 81:1679–1681, 1999.
Leigh JP, Kravitz RL, Schembri M, Samuels SJ, Mobley S. Physician career satisfaction across specialties. *Arch Intern Med* 162:1577–1584, 2002.

OTOLARYNGOLOGY

Otolaryngology, also known as ear, nose and throat (ENT), is a relatively small field that sees an extremely diverse patient population and performs a vast array of clinical and surgical procedures. However, its size belies the demand for these busy, specialized surgeons. Otolaryngologists enjoy some of the best aspects of both surgery and clinical medicine. Although the primary care specialties might take over allergy treatment as well as simple procedures such as tympanotomy, ENT physicians will continue to play key roles in academics, ENT oncology, pediatric otolaryngology, and the growing fields of facial plastics and otologic implants. As of the 2006 Match, all otolaryngology programs have switched from the early Match to the regular Match and participate with both ERAS and the NRMP. Most ENT programs are five years and include a one-year internship that combines general surgery rotations with rotations such as emergency medicine, anesthesia, neurosurgery, and critical care medicine. A few of the more prestigious, heavily academic programs offer positions with another year or two for research, usually between the general surgery and ENT years. Many ENT graduates pursue fellowship training in one of a number of subspecialty fields, including head and neck surgery, laryngology, otology, neurotology, rhinology, pediatrics, and plastic and reconstructive surgery.

Match Numbers

Otolaryngology continues to be an extremely competitive specialty. Both supply and demand have been steady; in 2005 there were 429 applicants for 254 positions (see Figure 4-12A). In 2005, only three of the 254 spots were left unfilled, leading to a staggering fill rate of 98.8%. In fact, the fill rate has remained near 100% for more than ten years (see Figure 4-12B). The rate of

OTOLARYNGOLOGY

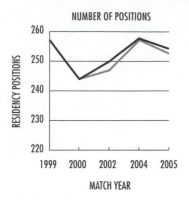

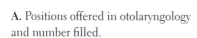

A. Positions offered in otolaryngology and number filled.

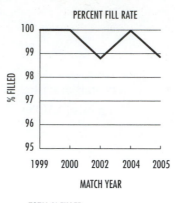

B. Percentage of otolaryngology positions filled on Match Day.

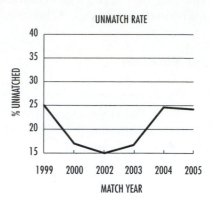

C. Percentage of U.S. seniors unmatched in otolaryngology on Match Day.

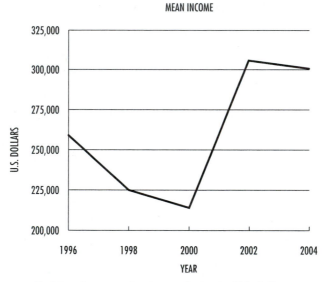

D. Mean income of otolaryngologists in U.S. dollars.

FIGURES 4-12A–D

U.S. seniors who did not match has dramatically increased over the past two years with unmatched rates in 2004 and 2005 of 24% and 23% respectively, up from 16% in 2003 (see Figure 4-12C). The average matched applicant scored 236 on the USMLE Step 1 exam. The average applicant in ENT submitted an average of 42 applications to receive nine interviews.

Application Tips

The keys to success in this highly competitive field are much the same as those in many of the other competitive specialties. Strong board scores are almost a prerequisite to a successful application. Students scoring below the 80th percentile on the USMLE Step 1 exam should seriously consider applying in another field in addition to ENT as a contingency. One recent study found that ENT matching success strongly correlates with high medical school GPAs (if available), high board scores, high class rank (if available), honors in both junior surgery and medicine, and AΩA selection. Some of the very competitive ENT programs suggest that applicants do an audition rotation at their hospital to increase their likelihood of being invited for an interview. In general, it's a good idea to do externships if you are aiming for specific programs where your application is less competitive than you'd like. Because there are only 100 or so programs in ENT and no more than a few spots available per program, you are also operating at a serious disadvantage if you have to apply in a particular geographic region.

As mentioned above, starting with the 2006 Match, all otolaryngology programs left the SF Match and began participating in the NRMP and using ERAS. Deadlines for applications will vary by program, with most being in October, but it is beneficial to submit your completed ERAS application as early as possible. The otolaryngology internship year is now under the control of the otolaryngology residency programs, and there is no longer a separate matching process for that year. The more programs you apply to, the higher the cost.

You are allowed to submit no more than four letters of recommendation via ERAS. The most balanced approach is to submit two to three letters from ENT faculty and one from a clinical attending from another major clerkship (e.g., medicine, OB/GYN, surgery). If you did ENT research, your research adviser can be one of your letter writers. If you did research outside of ENT, try to get two to three letters written by ENTs, with the third or fourth letter from your research adviser.

Interview Tips

The ENT interview season runs from mid-October into early February, with most interviews taking place in December and January. If you're offered an interview at one program, it would not hurt to call other programs you have approached in that geographic region to ask if they are willing to grant you an interview while you are in the area. Most ENT programs, however, have only two to three interview dates per season, so clustering interviews is often very difficult. Be ready to crisscross the country to get all the interviews you need, and prepare to spend anywhere from $3000 to $5000 on this process, from buying suits to paying travel expenses. It is generally cited that going to eight interviews is a good indication that you'll match; most applicants go to between 12 and 15 interviews.

An applicant will typically sit for six to eight interviews during the visit, each lasting 15 to 30 minutes—although it is not unheard of to have up to 13 half-hour interviews in one day. Interviews are generally held with one to two faculty members; panel interviews are relatively rare. This schedule usually includes an interview with the department chair, who in some cases is also the program director. During the interview, emphasize those strengths and interests which are most compatible with the philosophy of the particular program. It is also a good idea to highlight your academic and research interests when you are interviewed by the department chair even if the program is more clinically oriented. You should also feel free to drop names, assuming that the interview is going well and that you are well liked by the people whose names you drop. ENT is a small field in which anyone who's anyone knows everyone.

Everyone—from interviewers to tour guides to residents—will ask you if you have questions, and the right answer is always "yes." Even if you have asked all of your questions, it doesn't hurt to start repeating them. One way to do this is to open with "I have already asked most of my questions, but it's always nice to get a different perspective." You will be surprised by the extent to which perspectives within a single department can differ.

If asked to perform at an interview, remain calm, cool, and collected.

Some interviews may include a practical session in which you may be asked to suture, tie, carve soap, produce differential diagnoses, or identify radiologic landmarks. These types of interviews are, however, becoming exceedingly rare. Generally, the main point of these exercises is not to test your knowledge base but rather to see how you think under and deal with pressure. The best information on a particular program's interview style can be garnered from people who have already interviewed with that program; if you share your interview experiences, most other applicants will give you the skinny on places they have been. The best way to prepare for the unknown is to keep a case presentation ready for discussion. This is fair game and may be requested several times during the course of the interview season, even during the most benign interview sessions.

Note that if you are a competitive candidate, programs may try to ask you how you are ranking them. If a program is *not* your top choice, tell the interviewer(s) that you regard their program highly but cannot, in fairness, make that decision until you have finished your interviews. If the program does turn out to be one of your top choices, feel free to mention that in your follow-up thank-you letter. Programs may call you when most interviews have concluded to see if you have any questions. This is one semilegal way they can let you know they are interested in your application. Be honest with them, but also remain aware that you are not the only one they have contacted.

For More Info . . .

- Baylor University has a great Web site with links to most other programs: www.bcm.tmc.edu/oto/others.html.

- Other contacts include the following:

  American Academy of Otolaryngology—Head and Neck Surgery (AAO-HNS)
  One Prince Street
  Alexandria, VA 22314
  (703) 836-4444
  www.entnet.net

  American Academy of Facial Plastic and Reconstructive Surgery
  310 South Henry Street
  Alexandria, VA 22314
  (703) 299-9291
  (800) 332-FACE
  www.facial-plastic-surgery.org

American Board of Otolaryngology (ABOto)
3050 Post Oak Boulevard, Suite 1700
Houston, TX 77056
(713) 850-0399
www.aboto.org

Association for Research in Otolaryngology
www.aro.org

References

Calhoun KH, Hokanson JA, Bailey BJ. Predictors of residency performance: a follow-up study. *Otolaryngol Head Neck Surg* 116(6 Pt 1):647–651, 1997.

Kay DJ, Lucente FE. Otolaryngology residents' objectives in entering the workforce. *Laryngoscope* 112(10):1766–1768, 2002.

PATHOLOGY

The pathologist has long been known as the "doctor's doctor." One of the most traditional fields in medicine, pathology is the study of the mechanisms and manifestations of disease at a tissue level. The manner in which pathology is practiced has evolved dramatically from both a scientific and an economic perspective. The recent explosion in biomedical technology, especially in the area of genetics, has had a profound effect on the field. At the same time, the growing complexity of diagnostic tests has increased the governmental paperwork that is required to pay for such tests. As a result, specialists currently in the workforce find that they must work longer hours for the same pay. Furthermore, private practices are not hiring as many pathologists, especially in large urban centers, as these markets are brutally oversaturated. More residents are therefore delaying graduation from their training programs, choosing instead to acquire more distinctive fellowship skills in efforts to make themselves more desirable to potential employers. Many are also choosing research as an alternative to hospital practice. It would appear that the trend of decreasing job opportunities in pathology will continue in the near future, leading to many unemployed or underemployed pathologists.

Becoming board certified in either anatomic or clinical pathology requires a minimum of four years. Entering students should look at combined programs that offer a five-year residency covering both types of pathology, giving you a sort of "bilingual" appeal. If you are certified in only one specialty, you might be limited to working in large hospitals that can afford to employ separate specialists.

Pathology training is relatively flexible as long as the resident completes the core rotations required for board certification, such as surgical pathology, cytopathology, autopsy, and subspecialty rotations particular to each emphasis. He or she is then free to take elective courses, conduct research, or acquire further training in a specialized area of interest, such as forensic pathology.

Match Numbers

Despite its improved recognition, the field of pathology still suffers from a shortage of qualified applicants. Over the past two years, the number of positions offered by pathology programs has increased by 18% (see Figure 4-13A).

PATHOLOGY

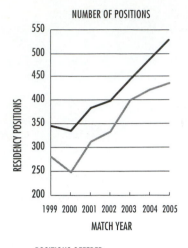

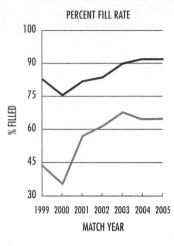

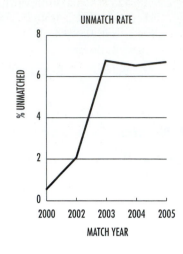

A. Positions offered in pathology and number filled.

B. Percentage of pathology positions filled on Match Day.

C. Percentage of U.S. seniors unmatched in pathology on Match Day.

FIGURES 4-13A–C

In the same time period, the number of positions filled has also increased. In 2002, only 333 of the 398 positions offered, or 83.6%, were filled through the NRMP Match (see Figures 4-13A and B). The fill rate increased to 90% in 2003 and held steady at 91% in 2004–2005. In general, students are usually able to match into the pathology program of their choice. Given the possible decline in job prospects, pathology programs are currently trying to find the ideal number of residency positions—i.e., a sufficient number to get residents' scut work done, yet not too many to risk leaving residents unemployed at graduation.

Application Tips

Because training programs in pathology have different emphases, it is important for you to find a program that matches your career goals. This is especially true for combined clinical and anatomic pathology programs, which may be strong in only one department. After you select your emphasis, the next step is to demonstrate your desire to enter pathology to the programs of your choice. A strong evaluation in the senior elective, accompanied by solid letters of recommendation (with at least one from a pathologist), is essential in this process. Many programs use their own application forms in place of the Universal Application supplied by the NRMP; however, this practice is waning.

Interview Tips

Given the less-than-glamorous image of pathology, most interviewers will be extremely curious to know why you are interested in the field. So be prepared to answer questions about your particular interests, any research background you possess, or any plans you might have for your future career. Interviews often last roughly 30 minutes, with three to six interviews a day depending on whether you are applying to the combined or the single program. In general, pathology interviews are relaxed, and only occasionally are tough questions asked. Expect to answer some questions about your postresidency plans, such as research, extra training, or going straight into private practice.

Pathology is a field in which a strong applicant is virtually assured the ability to write his or her own ticket to whatever residency he or she desires. However, this job market does have some potential pitfalls as well. Given the declining numbers of applicants over the years, pathology program directors, under increasing pressure to fill their programs, have resorted to "aggressive inquiry" tactics. In pathology more than in any other field, applicants may also be pressured by curious and sometimes overbearing program directors to disclose where they will rank a particular program. These negotiations, while strictly forbidden by the NRMP, can often lead a program director to offer an applicant a position "out of the Match." This practice is discussed in Chapter 12 of this book. Read the relevant section in that chapter and enter into any out-of-match deals with extreme caution.

It's a buyer's market in pathology, so shop carefully!

For More Info . . .

- *Student Information Packet.* This free packet includes several articles and a slick brochure about career opportunities in pathology. The College of American Pathologists (CAP) also produces a promotional video that it lends out at no cost. To receive an information packet or borrow the video, call or write:

  College of American Pathologists
  325 Waukegan Road
  Northfield, IL 60093
  (800) 323-4040
  www.cap.org

- American Society for Clinical Pathology (ASCP)
  2100 West Harrison Street
  Chicago, IL 60612-3798
  (312) 738-1336
  (800) 621-4142
  www.ascp.org

References

Alexander CB. Trends in pathology graduate medical education. *Hum Pathol* 32(7):671–676, 2001.
Bryant J. Underemployment: another aspect of the oversupply in pathology. *Hum Pathol* 30(9):1118–1119, 1999.
Kent JA. A tale of two systems: pathology resident recruitment in and out of the National Resident Matching Program. *Hum Pathol* 32(7):677–679, 2001.

Similar to internal medicine, pediatric programs are also divided into categorical and primary care programs. The categorical programs are geared more toward inpatient care with ample opportunity to explore subspecialty options, while primary care focuses more on general pediatrics. Pursuing a primary care track will not close the door on future subspecialty training.

Pediatricians enjoy developing relationships with their young patients as they grow up. Unlike family physicians, pediatricians can evaluate the whole family without assuming responsibility for each member's medical care. Today the field is seeing more routine procedures and well-child care done by nurse practitioners, physician assistants, and family practitioners, but this means that pediatricians can focus on the care of the seriously ill. Nevertheless, general pediatrics is tending to be more and more office based and increasingly oriented toward group practice. Career satisfaction tends to be higher than in other primary care fields. About 30–40% of graduates do subspecialty training, some after years of primary care practice (see Table 4-3). The trend in residency training favors increased ambulatory care, and many programs have trouble keeping up their inpatient census.

Pediatrics programs can be roughly classified according to their setting: children's versus non-children's hospitals. Children's hospitals have more pediatrics specialists available and in general offer more comprehensive training and education. In a children's hospital, everything is geared toward kids, from the intubating equipment in the ER to the wallpaper in the CT units. Children's hospitals also tend to be located in large cities and have more of a tertiary care focus. Good children's hospitals have affiliations with adult centers for delivery room experience.

By contrast, residencies in non-children's hospitals provide more interaction with faculty and house staff from other primary care specialties that involve children, such as family practice, OB/GYN, and internal medicine. These programs can be further categorized into community, university, and county/municipal settings. These are discussed in more detail in Chapter 6.

Match Numbers

The match rate for pediatrics programs has increased over the past three years, from 90% in 2002 to 92% in 2005. In the same period, the percentage of total matched residents who are U.S. graduates has also increased from 70% to 74% (see Figure 4-14B). Over the past three years the number of pediatrics positions has increased slightly, from 2341 to 2388 (see Figure 4-14A).

Application Tips

In the coming years, there will be excellent opportunities for both U.S. graduates and IMGs seeking positions in pediatrics. Since the quality of programs varies and some smaller programs may have difficulty providing adequate pathology, it is the applicant who must carefully decide where to apply. It goes without saying that your personal statement and CV should emphasize any involvement you might have with children, community or public health care, or volunteer activity. As in the other primary care specialties, the type of individual you are and your long-term goals will provide fodder for question-and-answer sessions.

Table 4-3. Pediatric Subspecialty Fellowships

Adolescent medicine

Developmental-behavioral pediatrics

Neonatal-perinatal medicine

Pediatric cardiology

Pediatric critical care medicine

Pediatric emergency medicine

Pediatric endocrinology

Pediatric gastroenterology

Pediatric hematology/oncology

Pediatric infectious diseases

Pediatric nephrology

Pediatric pulmonology

Pediatric rheumatology

Pediatric sports medicine

PEDIATRICS

NUMBER OF POSITIONS

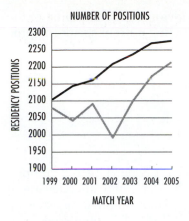

- **—** POSITIONS OFFERED
- **—** POSITIONS FILLED

A. Positions offered in pediatrics and number filled.

PERCENT FILL RATE

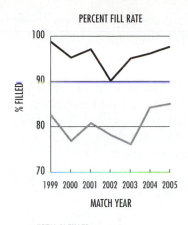

- **—** TOTAL % FILLED
- **—** U.S. % FILLED

B. Percentage of pediatrics positions filled on Match Day.

UNMATCH RATE

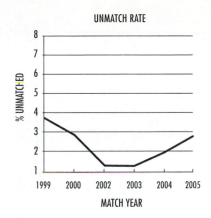

C. Percentage of U.S. seniors un-matched in pediatrics on Match Day.

MEAN INCOME

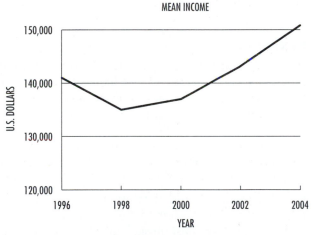

D. Mean income of pediatricians in U.S. dollars.

FIGURES 4-14A–D

Interview Tips

Most interviews for pediatrics programs are scheduled from late November through January. The interview day typically runs from 8 a.m. to 3 p.m. Expcct two to four interview sessions, each 20 to 45 minutes in length. Interviews in this specialty are generally low key and nonconfrontational. In addition to having the qualities typically desired in all house officers, you must package yourself as an individual who interacts well with parents and children. Good interpersonal skills are a must. Remember that most of your interviewers are parents themselves.

- *Pediatrics Information Packet.* In addition to giving a general profile of the specialty, this packet includes fact sheets detailing current socioeconomic statistics on pediatrics practice. To receive this information for free, call or write:

  American Academy of Pediatrics (AAP)
  141 Northwest Point Boulevard
  Elk Grove Village, IL 60007
  (847) 434-4000
  www.aap.org

- *Selecting a Pediatric Residency: An Employment Guide.* This is a comprehensive, step-by-step guide to selecting, applying to, and interviewing at pediatrics residency programs. It also discusses family and marriage considerations, employment issues such as contract and salary guidelines, and certification licensing requirements. It is available to medical students for $5 plus shipping costs. To order, call or write:

  AAP Publications Department
  P.O. Box 747
  Elk Grove Village, IL 60009-0927
  (888) 227-1770

References

Bradford BJ. Pediatric career choices. *Pediatrics* 110:647–648, 2002.

Pan RJ, Cull WL, Brotherton SE. Pediatric residents' career intentions: data from the leading edge of the pediatric workforce. *Pediatrics* 109:182–188, 2002.

Shelov SP, Burg FD. The pediatric residency match: a worrisome horizon. *Ambul Pediatr* 2:417–418, 2002.

PHYSICAL MEDICINE AND REHABILITATION

Physical medicine and rehabilitation (PM&R), also known as physiatry, is a relatively new and exciting field concerned with the diagnosis, evaluation, and treatment of musculoskeletal diseases and of patients with limited function secondary to injury, impairment, and disabilities. Physiatrists may specialize via fellowship in sports medicine and rehabilitation of sports injuries, work with patients with brain injury, or perform interventional pain management and electromyographic (EMG) procedures. They also care for patients with acute and chronic pain and musculoskeletal problems such as back and neck pain, pinched nerves, and fibromyalgia. Physiatrists are often involved in treating patients who have had major catastrophic events resulting in paraplegia, quadriplegia, traumatic brain injury, strokes, or orthopedic injury. They also treat neurological disorders such as multiple sclerosis, polio, and amyotrophic lateral sclerosis (ALS).

Physiatrists aim to restore function by taking a holistic approach toward patient diagnosis and treatment and considering the spectrum of physical, social, psychological, and vocational function. They are able to make and maintain relationships with their patients and see a wide variety of patient problems. They enjoy a comfortable lifestyle, often with minimal or no night calls. These attributes have led to PM&R residency becoming more popular and satisfying as a specialty. Some physiatrists may have broad practices, but the newer trend is to specialize in single areas such as pediatric rehabilitation, sports medicine, geriatric medicine, EMG and nerve conduction studies, and brain injury rehabilitation.

Physiatrists may treat patients individually or as consultants, or more commonly they coordinate patient care as leaders of a comprehensive team, including nurses, pain specialists, rehabilitation technicians, prosthetic experts, sports physiotherapists, neuropsychologists, and occupational and physical therapists. For example, a physiatrist treating a patient paralyzed from the neck down after a driving accident would assess the injury with a multidisciplinary team and plan the course of rehabilitation. Another example of a patient who might be seen by a physiatrist is a football player who tore his ACL and underwent surgery. The physiatrist, who may also be one of the team's sports physicians, would coordinate the rehabilitation thereafter with the goal of restoring maximal function.

There are more than 7000 trained physiatrists practicing in the United States. Residency training consists of one year in a transitional or preliminary program, followed by three years in a PM&R residency. Some institutions offer a four-year program that includes the internship, while others combine their programs with internal medicine and pediatrics. Fellowships are available in sports medicine and musculoskeletal rehabilitation, pain management, spinal cord injury/brain injury, pediatric rehabilitation, EMG, and interventional pain management.

Match Numbers

PM&R is growing in popularity (see Figures 4-15A–C) because it offers the physician the chance to practice holistic medicine, emphasizes building a re-

PM&R

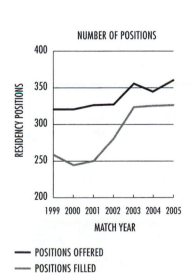

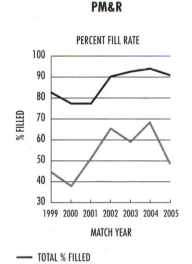

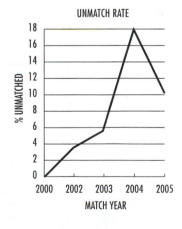

A. Positions offered in PM&R and number filled.

B. Percentage of PM&R positions filled on Match Day.

C. Percentage of U.S. seniors unmatched in PM&R on Match Day.

FIGURES 4-15A–C

lationship with the patient, and is associated with a very comfortable lifestyle. In addition, the use of more modern techniques, such as fluoroscopy, is making the field more exciting, particularly in the areas of sports medicine and interventional pain management. There are 80 accredited programs in the United States. Residency training at the top-tier programs can be very competitive, and only outstanding applicants with good scores, research experience, and strong LORs are granted interviews.

Application Tips

PM&R residency programs are imbalanced in the sense that the top programs are extremely competitive, while the rest of the programs are progressively less competitive. This disparity offers both U.S. graduates and IMGs many opportunities to match in good to very good programs. Programs vary greatly, especially in terms of the relative amount of inpatient rehabilitation training, musculoskeletal medicine, EMG training, and outpatient rehabilitation medicine that is offered. Some programs also incorporate a year of electives and research opportunities. Applicants should investigate these options closely and try to match them with their own preferences. It is best to pursue electives at the program(s) of choice before making a final decision.

Interview Tips

The applicant should show some understanding of the field to demonstrate a strong interest. At the top-rated programs, research experience and electives can make the difference. Expect three to four interviews of 15 to 30 minutes each. Interviewers generally take a relaxed approach and are usually very interested in the applicant's reason for choosing PM&R. Opportunities for research and specialized electives vary greatly among programs, and the interview is a good opportunity to obtain more specific information.

References

Braddom RL, Crawford J, DeLisa JA, Heilman D. Analysis of current practices in recruitment of residents for physical medicine and rehabilitation. *Am J Phys Med Rehabil* 77(4):317–325, 1998.

De Lisa JA, Jain SS, Campagnolo D, McCutcheon PH. Selecting a physical medicine and rehabilitation residency. *Am J Phys Rehabil* 71(2):72–76, 1992.

Millis SR, Campagnolo DI, Kirshblum S, Elovic E, Jain SS, DeLisa JA. Improving resident research in physical medicine and rehabilitation: impact of a structured training program. *J Spinal Cord Med* 27(5): 428–433, 2004.

Smith J, Krabak BJ, Malanga GA, Moutvic MA. Musculoskeletal education in physical medicine and rehabilitation residency programs. *Am J Phys Med Rehabil* 83(10): 785–790, 2004.

PSYCHIATRY

Although psychiatry attracts fewer U.S. graduates than there are residency slots, many outstanding students with interests in psychology or the social sciences are attracted to the field. The recent diagnostic and imaging advances in psychiatry are reigniting an intellectual interest in the field. Psychiatry is practiced in many different settings, with night call that is relatively light. The spectrum of disease varies with the patient population. The most recent national study finds career satisfaction to be relatively low. This may be due in part to reimbursement hassles, particularly in high-managed-care areas.

Residencies in psychiatry generally require a preliminary year, preferably in medicine, followed by three years of training in psychiatry. Some have a fourth year with emphasis in neurology or geriatrics. Depending on the program, training can emphasize either psychotherapy or the biological aspects of mental illness. For this reason, it is important to determine whether the orientation of a particular program matches your expectations and field of interest. Programs may vary in emphasis in fellowship areas such as child psychiatry, addiction, and geriatrics.

PSYCHIATRY

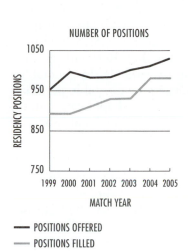

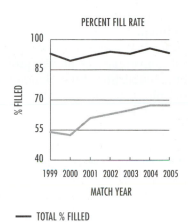

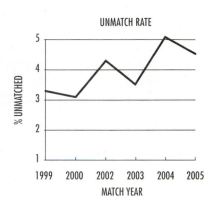

A. Positions offered in psychiatry and number filled.

B. Percentage of psychiatry positions filled on Match Day.

C. Percentage of U.S. seniors unmatched in psychiatry on Match Day.

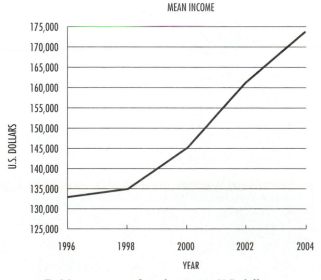

D. Mean income of psychiatrists in U.S. dollars.

FIGURES 4-16A–D

Match Numbers

Match rates in psychiatry have increased slightly over the past three years, from 94% in 2002 to 96% in 2005 (see Figure 4-16B). In 2002, only 60% of matched residents were U.S. medical school graduates, compared to 64% in 2005.

Application Tips

It is a reasonable assumption that strong interpersonal qualities and communication skills will be highly valued by program directors. Strong undergraduate backgrounds in psychology or experience working in a mental health field would also be evidence of commitment to psychiatry.

Interview Tips

Questions tend to probe the applicant's desire to enter psychiatry and his or her ability to interact with other people. There may be a variable called interpersonal culture that varies from one program to another. Residents evaluate the quality of a psychiatry residency program on this variable. In general, expect to meet psychiatrists who seek potential colleagues with stable personalities and good interpersonal skills. According to experienced applicants, an unspoken purpose of the interview is to rule out obvious psychological issues.

One purpose of the interview is to rule out obvious psychological issues.

For More Info . . .

■ *Directory of Psychiatric Residency Training Programs.* Although this directory is not updated as often as AMA-FREIDA, it has a more logical, user-friendly format. Information unique to the directory includes contact names and numbers for student electives, house staff contact names, and diagrams of a typical resident rotation schedule. The directory also offers general advice about residency applications. It is available at your psychiatry department or can be ordered for $25 with a student discount from:

> American Psychiatric Publishing, Inc.
> 1000 Wilson Blvd., Suite 1825
> Arlington, VA 22209
> (800) 368-5777
> www.appi.org

■ American Psychiatric Association (APA)
1000 Wilson Blvd., Suite 1825
Arlington, VA 22209-3901
(888) 35-PSYCH
(703) 907-7300
www.psych.org

■ American Academy of Child and Adolescent Psychiatry (AACAP)
3615 Wisconsin Avenue, N.W.
Washington, D.C. 20016
(202) 966-7300
www.aacap.org

References

Leigh JP, Kravitz RL, Schembri M, Samuels SJ, Mobley S. Physician career satisfaction across specialties. *Arch Intern Med* 162:1577–1584, 2002.

Yudowsky R, Elliott R, Schwartz A. Two perspectives on the indicators of quality in psychiatry residencies: program directors and residents. *Acad Med* 77(1):57–64, 2002.

RADIOLOGY

Radiology is a field that has grown tremendously over the last decade, thanks primarily to technological advances in imaging techniques. Radiologists continue to enjoy a good lifestyle, relatively high income (see Figure 4-17D), and flexible work hours. Practitioners in other fields, such as cardiology, gastroenterology, and urology, are performing many imaging-guided procedures that compete with the radiology workload. Nevertheless, radiologists are in increasing demand in many areas of the country. One recent study correlated the attractiveness of diagnostic radiology among students with the strength of the job market. Both were found to be very good. In choosing a residency program, students rate happiness of current residents, geographic location, and academic reputation as the most important factors influencing their selection process.

Training in radiology generally requires one preliminary year followed by four years of diagnostic radiology. The preliminary year can be satisfied through the completion of a transitional, surgical, or preliminary medicine year. The style of radiology training depends on the institution, but all institutions will cover the major imaging modalities, including nuclear medicine. Postresidency fellowships (one to two years) are offered in a wide variety of organ-based specialties, including neuroimaging, vascular/ interventional, mamography/women's imaging, body imaging, chest, and musculoskeletal. A number of modality-based fellowships, including computed tomography, magnetic resonance, ultrasonography, and nuclear medicine, are also available.

Match Numbers

Application to radiology residency programs remains extremely competitive. The number of positions offered has increased over the past three years from 920 in 2002 to 1018 in 2005 (see Figure 4-17A). Fill rates remain very high, reaching 98.5% in 2002 and 99.8% in 2003, and then dippling slightly to 95.6% in 2005 (see Figure 4-17B). In 2005, 972 of 1018 positions were filled in the Match, and 81% of matched applicants were U.S. medical graduates.

Application Tips

Strong evaluations in the senior clinical rotations, especially radiology, support the successful application. High board scores and excellent letters of recommendation by senior radiology faculty members are next in importance. Research experience or a technical background prior to entering medical school is also viewed favorably. As with other competitive specialties, early completion of application material is important. You will need to be well organized if you are to coordinate applications for both internship and residency positions. Students are usually advised to apply to 20 to 30 programs in order to obtain a comfortable 10 to 15 interviews.

Understand the differences between diagnostic radiology, nuclear medicine, and radiation oncology.

RADIOLOGY

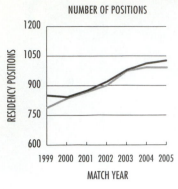

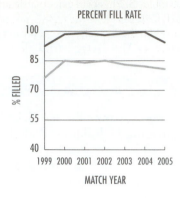

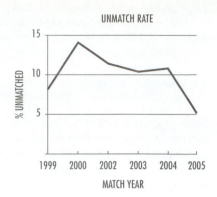

NUMBER OF POSITIONS

RESIDENCY POSITIONS

1200
1050
900
750
600

1999 2000 2001 2002 2003 2004 2005

MATCH YEAR

—— POSITIONS OFFERED
—— POSITIONS FILLED

A. Positions offered in radiology and number filled.

PERCENT FILL RATE

% FILLED

100
85
70
55
40

1999 2000 2001 2002 2003 2004 2005

MATCH YEAR

—— TOTAL % FILLED
—— U.S. % FILLED

B. Percentage of radiology positions filled on Match Day.

UNMATCH RATE

% UNMATCHED

15
10
5

1999 2000 2002 2003 2004 2005

MATCH YEAR

C. Percentage of U.S. seniors unmatched in radiology on Match Day.

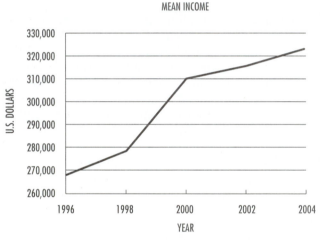

MEAN INCOME

U.S. DOLLARS

330,000
320,000
310,000
300,000
290,000
280,000
270,000
260,000

1996   1998   2000   2002   2004

YEAR

D. Mean income of radiologists in U.S. dollars.

FIGURES 4-17A–D

Interview Tips

Because of the small number of spots available, residency programs in radiology tend to offer interviews only to strong applicants in whom they are seriously interested. A candidate's visit typically includes two to five interviews, each 15 to 30 minutes in length. Interviews for radiology often tend to be relaxed, placing major emphasis on the applicant's reason for entering the field and interviewing at this particular institution. You might also be invited to attend a clinical case conference, but almost no one expects you to be able to read an x-ray on the spot. Quantifying a "good eye" in radiology is even harder than evaluating manual dexterity for a surgical field, so programs don't even try. During the interview sessions, it may be particularly important to assess resident working conditions and satisfaction, which vary significantly from one program to another.

For More Info . . .

■ *Career Information Packet.* This packet includes a brochure describing the field of radiology as well as several articles describing job prospects, average earnings, and practice characteristics. This information can be obtained free of charge by calling or writing:

American College of Radiology (ACR)
1891 Preston White Drive
Reston, VA 20191-4397
(703) 648-8900
(800) ACR-LINE
www.acr.org

References

Anzilotti K, Kamin DS, Sunshine JH, Forman HP. Relative attractiveness of diagnostic radiology: assessment with data from the National Residency Match Program and comparison with the strength of the job market. *Radiology* 221(1):87–91, 2001.

Pretorius ES, Hrung J. Factors that affect National Resident Matching Program rankings of medical students applying for radiology residency. *Acad Radiol* 9(1):75–80, 2002.

RADIATION ONCOLOGY

Radiation oncologists are an essential part of the multidisciplinary management of cancer patients, collaborating closely with other physicians. Radiation oncology uses radiation therapy in the treatment of patients with cancer and other diseases. The field is attractive to many because of its relatively easy lifestyle and minimal call duties. As a result, it is becoming more and more competitive.

A one-year internship either in internal medicine or as a transitional year is required for this specialty, followed by four years of residency in radiation oncology. A study published in 2001 found that directors' perceptions of the marketplace for radiation oncologists was very good. The quality of residents in radiation oncology programs was felt to be improving.

Match Numbers

The number of residency positions in this field has been increasing for the past several years, with 137 positions being offered through the NRMP in 2005 (see Figure 4-18A). The field has become increasingly competitive because it is seen by some as having a relatively easy lifestyle, and in 2005, 225 applicants applied for the available positions. In 2003, all 117 positions matched for a fill rate of 100%, and in both 2004 and 2005 fill rates remained above 98% (see Figure 4-18B). In 2005, 87% of those matched were U.S. graduates (see Figure 4-18B).

Application Tips

Given the increasing competitiveness of radiation oncology, applicants should do their best to have a strong application so as to increase their chances of matching. Strong letters of recommendation from internal medicine specialists, oncologists, and radiation oncologists are important. In addition, strong

RADIATION ONCOLOGY

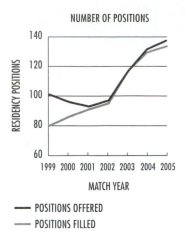

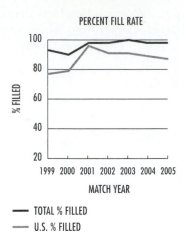

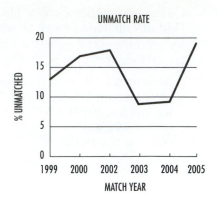

NUMBER OF POSITIONS

PERCENT FILL RATE

UNMATCH RATE

— POSITIONS OFFERED
— POSITIONS FILLED

— TOTAL % FILLED
— U.S. % FILLED

A. Positions offered in radiation oncology and number filled.

B. Percentage of radiation oncology positions filled on Match Day.

C. Percentage of U.S. seniors unmatched in radiation oncology on Match Day.

FIGURES 4-18A–C

research within the field of radiation oncology is extremely important, as are excellent board scores and clerkship grades.

Interview Tips

Interviews are usually conducted on an individual basis. Expect three to four interviews lasting approximately 30 minutes each. Students should express interest in caring for cancer patients and in the basic science on which the field is based. Lifestyle is usually a clear advantage in this field of medicine but should not be the major factor governing its selection. Opportunities for academic medicine and research pursuits may be limited in some programs. In the course of your discussions, make sure there are adequate staff to teach the basic science principles of the discipline.

For More Info . . .

- American College of Radiation Oncology (ACRO)
  4350 East West Highway, Suite 401
  Bethesda, MD 20814
  (301) 718-6515
  www.acro.org

- American Society for Therapeutic Radiology and Oncology (ASTRO)
  12500 Fair Lakes Circle, Suite 375
  Fairfax, VA 22033-3882
  (800) 962-7876
  (703) 502-1550
  www.astro.org

References

Bushee GR, Sunshine JH, Schepps B. The status of radiation oncology training programs and their graduates in 1999. *Int J Radiat Oncol Biol Phys* 49(1):133–1138, 2001.

Radiation Oncology Resident Training Working Group. Radiation oncology training in the United States: report from the Radiation Oncology Resident Training Working Group organized by the Society of Chairman of Academic Radiation Oncology Programs (SCAROP). *Int J Radiat Oncol Biol Phys* 45(1):153–161, 1999.

Zeman EM, Dynlacht JR, Rosenstein BS, Dewhirst MW. Toward a national consensus: teaching radiobiology to radiation oncology residents. *Int J Radiat Oncol Biol Phys* 54(3):861–872, 2002.

SURGERY

General surgery abounds with both positive and negative attributes, all of which influence students' thinking about a career in the field. The specialty boasts a number of benefits: the chance to apply technical and procedural skills to the quick resolution of medical problems; good doctor-patient relationships; and relatively high income (see Figure 4-19D). Drawbacks include long hours, rigorous training, increasing paperwork, and the intrusion of prickly nonclinical issues such as malpractice liability, government regulations, and third-party payers. The demanding work hours and culture seem to be especially tough on women, and the field consistently has more male applicants. However, with the instatement of the 80-hour workweek, this trend may not be as pronounced in the future. Generally, most surgeons remain highly satisfied with their work, notwithstanding the changes they have been forced to make in their practices to accommodate HMOs and other complications.

Surgical residencies require a minimum of five years of training, with some programs requiring as many as three additional research years. These often come in the middle or latter portion of the residency, at a time when residents can also moonlight. A general surgery residency is also the way to enter into a variety of surgical subspecialties. Subspecialty training includes critical care, hand, pediatric, plastic, cardiothoracic, vascular, and trauma surgery.

Match Numbers

Surgery has historically been very competitive, and the competition has increased over the past couple of years since the 80-hour workweek went into effect. In 2005, 1044 of the 1051 positions available were filled through the NRMP on Match Day, resulting in a 99.3% fill rate (see Figures 4-19A and B). For the past several years U.S. graduates have filled 80–85% of the offered positions (Figure 4-19B). Both the number of positions offered and the number filled have remained relatively stable; however, the unmatched rate of students dropped from 5.4% in 2002 to around 17% in 2005 (see Figure 4-19C).

Application Tips

Surgeons are hands-on people; they know things by seeing them. Applicants are no different. General surgery, like many surgical subspecialties, places great currency in the acting subinternship. It is therefore strongly recommended that applicants who are examining competitive programs consider doing an away rotation at that location.

GENERAL SURGERY

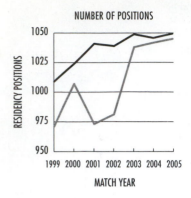

A. Positions offered in general surgery and number filled.

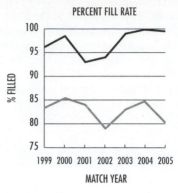

B. Percentage of general surgery positions filled on Match Day.

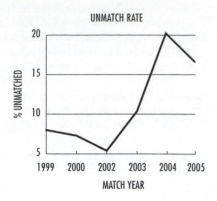

C. Percentage of U.S. seniors unmatched in general surgery on Match Day.

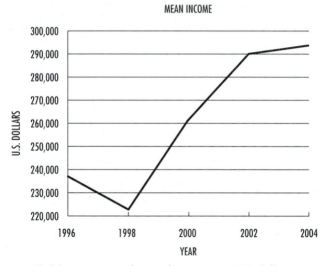

D. Mean income of general surgeons in U.S. dollars.

FIGURES 4-19A–D

Before applying, you should think about whether you would be happier in a clinical or a research-oriented program, bearing in mind that length of training varies from one type of program to the other. Most academic programs are seven years in length, and community programs are five years. Strong evaluations in the senior surgical rotations are generally essential to successful applications. The *pièce de résistance* would be a strong letter from the chief of surgery. Programs with an academic slant will definitely consider the applicant's research background fundamental to the evaluation process, whereas those with a clinical focus will attempt to determine the applicant's potential to be a good surgeon. In a recent retrospective study, the most important applicant attributes were found to be enthusiasm, work ethic, and ability.

For advice and connection purposes, it's always helpful to find a mentor who is well known in the field. As with other competitive residencies, early completion of application material is important. Although the desired number of applications depends on the applicant's quality, the average ranges from 15 to 20, with a goal of obtaining at least 10 to 12 interviews.

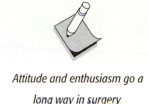

Attitude and enthusiasm go a long way in surgery.

Interview Tips

The field of surgery is infamous for having some of the most colorful personalities in medicine. However, while the brilliant attending transplant surgeon may well be revered for his skill and feared for his outbursts of temper, no one is looking for the latter quality in a resident. Although interview committees often have a good idea of how they are going to rank you before they even meet you, the interview is an essential part of the process, if only to eliminate interpersonally challenged applicants. Uniquely, surgical interview days are usually held on Saturdays, making it difficult for applicants to schedule more than one interview in a single trip. Interviews often consist of two to three sessions lasting 30 to 45 minutes each. Occasionally, an applicant is asked to present a clinical case or to discuss how to deal with the stress of a surgical residency. One should have a prepared answer to this latter question in particular. Interviews are often laid back, with little or no pimping. However, academic programs tend to opt for more pointed questions and may inquire about your research background as well as any current projects. Try to learn something about the program's reputation for research.

For More Info . . .

- Johansen K, Heimbach DM. *So You Want to Be a Surgeon: A Medical Student Guide to Finding and Matching with the Best Possible Surgery Residency.* This book includes a brief but very helpful discussion of surgical residency applications. The greater part of the book is devoted to descriptions of most of the surgery programs in the United States and Puerto Rico. The authors attempt to classify programs by the caliber of the house staff. The book can be accessed online at www.facs.org/residencysearch/. The book is also in some medical bookstores and can also be ordered for about $12 from:

    > Educational Clearinghouse
    > Department of Surgery
    > Southern Illinois University
    > School of Medicine
    > P.O. Box 19230
    > Springfield, IL 62794
    > (217) 785-3835

- *The Surgical Career Handbook.* This glossy booklet provides an overview of surgery and profiles its subspecialties. However, the information is often too general to be useful. This publication is available for $7 from:

    > American College of Surgeons (ACS)
    > 633 North Saint Clair Street
    > Chicago, IL 60611
    > (312) 202-5000
    > www.facs.org

References

Dunnington GL, Williams RG. Addressing the new competencies for residents' surgical training. *Acad Med* 78(1):14–21, 2003.

Gilbart MK, Cusimano MD, Regehr G. Evaluating surgical resident selection procedures. *Am J Surg* 18(3):221–225, 2001.

Mayer KL, Perez RV, Ho HS. Factors affecting choice of surgical residency training program. *J Surg Res* 98(2):71–75, 2001.

TRANSITIONAL-YEAR PROGRAM

For those on a quest for a flexible internship, transitional-year programs (TYPs) continue to be a popular choice. In contrast to the preliminary medicine or preliminary surgery years, transitional internships allow for exposure to many other fields, such as OB/GYN, EM, orthopedics, pediatrics, and anesthesia as well as traditional medicine and surgery. Transitional internships consist of multiple rotations through different departments. The length of each rotation and the type of work involved are usually extremely flexible and can be tailored to each individual's need. Some programs will have certain required core rotations that must be satisfied. In general, however, these requirements are minimal and can be easily fulfilled. The variety of experience in TYPs is ideal for anyone entering a residency such as EM, in which a wide base of knowledge is desirable.

Other students take a TYP because they're undecided on a specialty, but this can prove to be a difficult undertaking. By the time your year starts, the application process is already upon you. In addition, finding time for interviews during the year can be impossible. So make sure you reach an understanding with the program director/chief resident regarding the time you will need to apply and interview. If you can't take sufficient time off, it may be preferable to take a year off for research or an MPH.

Match Numbers

Although TYPs were not considered competitive in the past, the number of unmatched students has risen dramatically over the past several years (see Figure 4-20C). The number of positions offered by programs has declined over time from 1337 in 1994 to 1012 in 2005 (see Figure 4-20A). In 2005, 967 of 1017 positions, or 95% of all available positions, were filled (see Figure 4-20B). The number of positions filled by IMGs decreased from 25% in 1996 to approximately 10% in 2005 (see Figure 4-20B).

Application Tips

As with most internship programs, the competitiveness of the TYP depends on the reputation of the institution and on the flexibility of the program. Applicants should have strong clinical evaluations, good letters of recommendation, and convincing reasons for seeking a transitional internship. Board scores tend to be less important except at highly prestigious institutions. Early submission of application material is important. Despite the February date posted by many programs, the recommended deadline is early November.

TRANSITIONAL YEAR

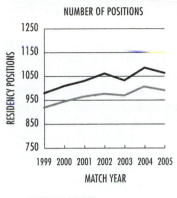

NUMBER OF POSITIONS

— POSITIONS OFFERED
— POSITIONS FILLED

A. Positions offered in TYPs and number filled.

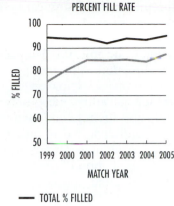

PERCENT FILL RATE

— TOTAL % FILLED
— U.S. % FILLED

B. Percentage of TYP positions filled on Match Day.

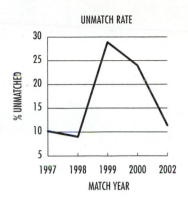

UNMATCH RATE

C. Percentage of U.S. seniors unmatched in TYPs on Match Day.

FIGURES 4-20A–C

Interview Tips

Interviews are casual and are even optional for some programs. The applicant will usually be scheduled for two or three sessions lasting 30 minutes each. Questions attempt to ascertain the candidate's ability to fit in with the program, desire for a transitional residency, and long-term plans. Interviews for TYPs should center on how the immediate needs of the program and long-term goals of the applicant can be mutually beneficial.

For More Info . . .

■ *Transitional Year Program Directory.* More popularly known as the "Purple Book," this annually updated directory is available at your student affairs office. You can order your own copy by calling or writing:

> Association for Hospital Medical Education
> Council of Transitional Year Program Directors
> 419 Beulah Road
> Pittsburgh, PA 15235
> (412) 244-9302
> (866) 617-4780
> www.ahme.org

■ Additional information may be obtained from:

> Mary Catherine Nace, MD
> Chair of the Council of Transitional Year Program Directors
> Walter Reed Army Medical Center
> 13911 Crest Hill Lane
> Silver Spring, MD 20905
> (301) 879-1918

Urology is the medical and surgical specialty that deals with disorders of the male and female urinary tract and the male reproductive organs. Urologists see patients with kidney, ureter, bladder, prostate, urethra, and male genital structure disorders and injuries. They also investigate and treat infertility and male sexual dysfunction. Although generally classified as a surgical specialty, urology also encompasses knowledge of internal medicine, pediatrics, gynecology, and other specialties. Diagnostic procedures are routinely performed in this specialty and include endoscopic, percutaneous, and open surgery to treat congenital and acquired disorders of the reproductive and urinary systems and related structures. Urologists enjoy seeing a variety of patients and appreciate the combination of medicine and surgery in one specialty. As a result, urology is a popular and competitive field despite the rigors of its residency training.

Residency training involves one to two years of training in a general surgery program, followed by at least three to four years in a urology training program. The urology residency program is carried out under the auspices of the American Urological Association (AUA). Some urology programs also use the Electronic Residency Application Service (ERAS).

A paper published in 2000 summarized a study in which the behaviors and attitudes of both applicants and program directors in the urology match were evaluated. The results suggested a need to improve the ethical behavior of participants in the process. The study found, for example, that applicants were sometimes inappropriately asked how they would rank programs, while others were asked questions about marital status and intent to have children.

Match Numbers

Urology is an extremely competitive specialty. The number of positions offered by programs has remained relatively constant over the past several years, between 220 and 240 (see Figure 4-21A). In 2005, all 232 positions were filled in the Match, and in 2004 only four positions went unfilled (see Figures 4-21A and B). In previous years, the total fill rate was similarly high, often above 99% (see Figure 4-21B). As expected, there is a high rate of unmatched applicants each year, with 22% of U.S. seniors going unmatched in 2005 and as many as 29% in 2003 (see Figure 4-21C). Only 16% of IMGs matched in 2005, and this was down from 25% in 2004.

Application Tips

Urology applications go through an early match. It is recommended that students submit their applications as soon as possible. Although the deadline for applications is usually November or December, applications should be mailed by October. Factors that will make your application stronger include AΩA status; high USMLE scores; a high GPA, particularly with respect to medicine and surgery clerkship grades; and a recommendation from the chief of urology. Research or special experience in urology provides a competitive advantage. The AUA reports that the average number of applications per individual was 41.2 and the average number of interviews 10.2.

UROLOGY

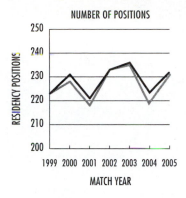

NUMBER OF POSITIONS

— POSITIONS OFFERED
— POSITIONS FILLED

A. Positions offered in urology and number filled.

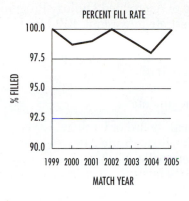

PERCENT FILL RATE

— TOTAL % FILLED

B. Percentage of urology positions filled on Match Day.

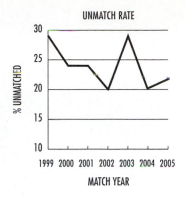

UNMATCH RATE

C. Percentage of U.S. seniors un-matched in urology on Match Day.

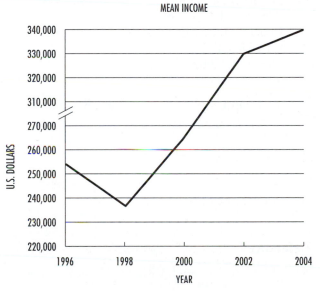

MEAN INCOME

D. Mean income of urologists in U.S. dollars.

FIGURES 4-21A–D

Interview Tips

Interviews may be conducted on a group or individual basis and are usually informal and relaxed. There are usually two to three interviews lasting 30 to 45 minutes each. Interviewers attempt to ascertain your personality and whether or not it is compatible with theirs. Applicants should be prepared to describe how they acquired their interest in urology. Expect direct questions about your interest in the clinical and/or research aspects of the program to which you are applying.

For More Info . . .

- Listing of Accredited Urology Programs
  Administrative Assistant, RRC for Urology
  Accreditation Council for Graduate Medical Education
  515 North State Street, Suite 2000
  Chicago, IL 60610
  (312) 755-5000
  www.acgme.org

- American Board of Urology
  2216 Ivy Road, Suite 210
  Charlottesville, VA 22903
  (434) 979-0059
  www.abu.org

- American Urological Association Headquarters
  1120 North Charles Street
  Baltimore, MD 21201
  (410) 727-1100
  www.auanet.org

- American Urological Association Office of Education
  2425 West Loop South, Suite 333
  Houston, TX 77027-4207
  (800) 282-7077
  (713) 622-2700
  www.auanet.org

- American Urological Association Residency Matching Program
  2425 West Loop South, Suite 333
  Houston, TX 77027-4207
  (800) 282-7077, ext. 86
  (713) 622-2700, ext. 86
  Vacancy hotline: (800) 282-7077, ext. 88
  www.auanet.org

References

Andriole DA, Schechtman KB, Ryan K, Whelan A, Diemer K. How competitive is my surgical specialty? *Am J Surg* 184(1):1–5, 2002.

Kerfoot BP, Mitchell ME, Novick AC. Grappling with the evaluation of clinical competencies: a view from the Residency Review Committee for Urology. *Urology* 60(2):223–224, 2002.

Teichman JM, Anderson KD, Dorough MM, Stein CR, Optenberg SA, Thompson IM. The urology residency matching program in practice. *J Urol* 163(6):1878–1887, 2000.

CHAPTER 5

International Medical Graduates and the Match Process

IMGs continue to play an important role in providing health care for Americans.

INTRODUCTION

An international medical graduate (IMG) can be broadly defined as anyone who has graduated from a medical school outside the United States, Canada, or Puerto Rico. IMGs have been divided into U.S. citizen IMGs and non-U.S. citizen IMGs. The group as a whole represents roughly one-quarter of both U.S. residents and U.S. practicing physicians. The provision of medical care and the filling of residency programs in the United States have always relied heavily on applications from IMGs, who continue to play an important role in providing health care for Americans in both urban and rural areas. The number of residency spots offered in the United States exceeds the number of graduates from U.S. medical schools by roughly 30%. These spots must be filled, and residency programs often look to IMGs for this purpose (see Table 5-1).

In 2004, about 215,900 IMGs received medical degrees from more than 130 countries, representing about 24% of the approximately 910,700 physicians practicing in the United States. There are differences and similarities in the demographics of IMGs as a whole in comparison to U.S. medical graduates. For example, more than half of all IMGs train in primary care, as compared to only one-third of U.S. graduates. Internal medicine has been the most popular primary specialty with IMGs, followed by anesthesiology, psychiatry, and pediatrics. The IMG population has increased by more than 100,000 physicians since the 1970s, predominantly in these four specialties. In terms of total physician counts in the United States, IMGs accounted for approximately 21% of the total in the 1980s and currently represent 24% of the total physician count. The states with the highest concentrations of IMGs are New Jersey and New York, with nearly 40% IMG physicians. Illinois and Florida also have a large number of IMGs, who account for approximately 30% of all physicians. A recent study on initial practice locations for IMGs found that they were more likely to be located in the same state where they received their GME training and less likely to choose a market with more stringent licensure requirements. Furthermore, this study showed that IMG physicians were more likely to locate in markets with established higher proportions of IMG physicians, suggesting that networks among established IMGs played a role.

A study in *JAMA* described some changes that have taken place in the demographics of IMGs in the United States. Specifically, this study found that between 1995 and 2001, the number of IMGs initiating the accreditation process in the United States was reduced by 46%. This change was thought to

TABLE 5-1. IMGs in the Match

APPLICANTS	2002	2003	2004	2005
U.S.-citizen IMGs	2029	1987	2015	2091
% U.S. citizens accepted	54	55	55	55
Non-U.S.-citizen IMGs	4556	5029	5671	5554
% non-U.S. citizens accepted	51	56	52	56

have resulted from the declining number of residency positions available in the United States. However, even with this precipitous drop in the number of IMGs seeking certification, the authors concluded that the applicant pool continues to supply an ample number of capable individuals to fill U.S. residency positions.

Another study looking at board specialty certification among U.S. graduates and IMGs found that IMGs generally have lower board-certification rates than do U.S. graduates. A subgroup analysis showed that the non-U.S.-citizen IMGs had better certification rates than did U.S.-citizen IMGs. After the devastating terrorist attacks on September 11, 2001, the process of immigrating and obtaining visas has become more challenging. Taken together, these findings make it evident that IMGs who are applying to train in the United States must be armed not only with the medical skills and knowledge needed to be good doctors but also with a detailed understanding of the numerous steps required to gain residency and accreditation. These complicated steps are addressed in this chapter and elsewhere in this book.

As compared to U.S. graduates, the IMG has to go through a longer residency application process, which is followed by an interview process that may seem less friendly to IMGs. Indeed, some studies have shown that when comparing IMGs and U.S. medical graduates with similar skills and abilities, U.S. medical graduates were favored in the recruitment process for several reasons, including the pressure to rank U.S. graduates higher so as to avoid a reduced complement of U.S. medical graduates in the program. Despite this inequity, the overall process is streamlined to ensure that IMGs who match find little difference in quality among residents, whether they graduated from medical school in the United States or abroad.

IMGs must be armed with medical skills and knowledge, as well as a detailed understanding of the residency process.

THE GENERAL APPROACH

The financial, emotional, and time commitments required throughout the application and Match process is certainly an important factor for any applicant. IMGs face the added challenges of traveling from abroad, applying for visas, obtaining security clearances, and settling down in a new country. However, this objective is not impossible to realize as long as you are organized, use a stepwise approach, and keep your eyes on the prize: Match Day. A strong commitment and a resilient spirit are two of the most important ingredients for success during the matching process.

If you want to pursue postgraduate training in the United States, start planning while you are still in medical school. Usually, the best time is during the third or fourth year, when elective rotations are completed. The goal is to match the typical credentials of the U.S. medical graduate applicant. Most seniors in U.S. medical programs will have done electives in specialties corresponding to their desired residency. Some will also rotate at institutions where they will apply for residency positions. Hence, IMGs should try to do an elective at a U.S. institution in their specialty of choice, and this process must start early in the clinical years.

Your goal is to match or exceed the typical credentials of the U.S. medical graduate applicant.

An elective performed in the United States has many advantages:

■ Obtaining firsthand experience of U.S. clinical settings. It is extremely difficult to obtain clinical exposure in the United States once you are finished with medical school for medical/legal and insurance reasons.

- Creating a favorable impression with U.S. faculty and identifying potential future writers for letters of recommendation.
- Taking advantage of improved accessibility to some institutions where IMGs are more accepted as medical students.
- Improving the potential for interview offers at institutions where IMGs have previously performed electives.
- Applying for a visa to participate in elective rotations may make it easier to obtain one for residency, as some of the prerequisites may be the same.

Doing an elective in the United States has numerous advantages.

Obviously, doing an elective in the United States creates extra expenses that need to be budgeted for, such as airline tickets, visa costs, expenses for accommodation, in-country travel, and food during the interview process.

Even though there are many benefits to doing an elective in the United States as a medical student, it is by no means a requirement for success in the Match. Indeed, most IMGs have not done electives prior to arriving in the United States. For each IMG, the first step toward establishing a medical career in the United States is resolving the question: "When should I go to the United States?" If you are not able to participate in an elective in the United States during medical school, this question has an easy answer. All who wish to be accredited by the U.S. board in their specialty of choice must do all their training, from PGY-1 (internship year) onward, in the United States.

Deciding when to go to the United States for medical training is the first key question you must answer.

It is important to get in touch with the Educational Commission for Foreign Medical Graduates (ECFMG) for the application materials. Their Web site (www.ecfmg.org) has information on the application and a time line of events with application deadlines for United States Medical Licensing Examination (USMLE) Steps. (Information on these exams is provided later in this chapter.)

After making the choice to train in the United States, it is important to gather information on individual programs in your desired specialty throughout the United States. You may be able to get more information via specific program coordinators or through official program Web sites. An important source of information is current doctors or residents in training. For example, Web-based forums may give you better insight into individual programs. Communication with individual programs may also reveal lists of residency program alumni who do not mind being contacted.

The next big step is to prepare for the USMLE exams. It is usually best to take these exams during or immediately after medical school, when the knowledge is freshest in your mind. Whereas high scores on the USMLE do not necessarily grant the IMG a place in residency, such scores can help to ensure good interviews, thus opening more doors in the Match process. Most of the USMLE exams can be taken in your home country (more information can be found on the ECFMG Web site). Currently, the Step 2 Clinical Skills (CS) exam is administered at selected centers in the United States only. Once you have completed the exams, you can apply for the residency of your choice via the Match.

One of the most troubling questions for IMGs is whether their USMLE score will be good enough to secure interviews in the United States. The section that follows has strategies to enhance your chances as an IMG. However, even IMGs with near-perfect scores have matched at less desirable residency locations, while those with average scores have matched well due to research experience (and possibly publications), U.S. elective experience, and strong letters of recommendation. The bottom line is while USMLE scores may serve as a numeric point for screening applicants, many other factors determine one's success during the matching process.

It is possible to do a residency in your home country and then come to the United States for specialty training. If you wish to be licensed by the U.S.-based board in your specialty, however, you must begin and finish postgraduate training in the United States. Once you have decided that you wish to enter the U.S. Match, it will be worth your while to consider the specialty in which you are going to apply. As mentioned above, many IMGs apply to primary care residencies because it is widely perceived that IMGs have a higher success rate in this field. In fact, the numbers do support this approach. Recently, one in four family medicine residents was an IMG, whereas only 2% of ophthalmology residents were IMGs. Although these numbers clearly do not prevent IMGs from applying in other fields, they do offer an indication of where IMGs have historically achieved the most success (see Chapter 4 for details on your specialty). At the same time, the notion that IMGs perform at the bottom of every field is not substantiated by current data. For example, a recent article from the *Annals of Internal Medicine* observed that IMGs have outperformed U.S. medical graduates on internal medicine in-training exams.

IMGs have outperformed U.S. medical graduates on internal medicine in-training exams.

Once you have chosen the field in which you wish to match, you will find that the process of applying to the programs is much like that for U.S. medical graduates. The necessary components are listed in Table 5-2.

The USMLE

The USMLE Steps 1 through 3 are a set of medical exams that are designed to evaluate your readiness to enter the U.S. medical system. Directors of residency programs in the United States often have a difficult time comparing U.S. medical graduate applicants by virtue of the different grading schemes, requirements, and levels of competition found at various U.S. medical schools. Not surprisingly, many program directors also find that comparing IMGs to U.S. medical graduates or to one another is extremely challenging. The USMLE Steps provide at least one objective criterion against which to make such comparisons (see Table 5-3 for pass rates for first-time test takers). It is therefore essential that any IMG who is considering residency in the United States excel on all three Steps, and particularly on Step 1. Refer to *First Aid for the USMLE Step 1* and *First Aid for the USMLE Step 2 CK* for additional information and advice on this subject. Here are some key facts about the USMLE:

Don't feel singled out by the CS exam. The U.S. medical students have to take it, too!

- The USMLE Steps 1 and 2 CK are now administered exclusively by computer and are given on a continuous basis throughout the world.
- The test is administered to IMGs by the ECFMG rather than by the National Board of Medical Examiners (NBME).
- In order to register for the USMLE Step 1, you must first have taken the basic sciences coursework at your medical school.
- Registration for the USMLE Step 2 Clinical Knowledge (CK) and Clinical Skills (CS) exams also requires that you be within one year of graduation from your medical school.
- To be certified by ECFMG, international medical graduates must, among other requirements, pass a medical science examination. Obtaining a pass-

Testing performance is an important determinant of success in the Match for IMGs. Be prepared.

TABLE 5-2. **Steps in Your Application to Various Programs**

1. Have your school verify that you have completed the two years of basic science training.

2. Apply for and pass the United States Medical Licensing Examination (USMLE) Step 1.

3. Apply for and pass the USMLE Step 2 Clinical Knowledge (CK).

4. Graduate from medical school and obtain your degree.

5. Send a copy of your medical degree to the Educational Commission for Foreign Medical Graduates (ECFMGs).

6. Obtain a **current** ECFMG certificate.

7. Pass the USMLE Step 2 Clinical Skills (CS).

8. Send for an Electronic Residency Application Service (ERAS) application.

9. Register as an "independent applicant" with the National Resident Matching Program (NRMP).

10. Research and choose programs to apply to electronically through ERAS.

11. Obtain interview invitations and interview.

12. Rank programs through the NRMP.

13. Review visa options from various programs and begin your visa paperwork.

14. Review licensing requirements in each state in which you applied, and consider beginning licensing paperwork in your preferred state.

TABLE 5-4. **USMLE Step 2 CS Pass Rates***

U.S. students	96%
IMGs	83%

*From June 2004 through March 2005.

ing score on both Steps 1 and 2 CK currently fulfills this requirement for certification. You can take Step 1 or Step 2 CK in either order, provided you meet the eligibility requirements for these exams.

■ Step 2 CS replaced the Clinical Skills Assessment (CSA), formerly administered by the ECFMG. To register for Step 3, ECFMG certificate holders will have to have taken and passed either the CSA or the Step 2 CS. The CS exam is offered in five locations: Atlanta, Chicago, Houston, Los Angeles, and Philadelphia. The purpose of this test is for students to demonstrate the ability to collect and analyze data and to communicate well with patients. (See Table 5-4 for CS results.)

■ Registration for the USMLE Step 3 is possible only after you have completed between one and three years of residency or if you are a physician not participating in the Match.

■ You will need to the pass Step 3 if you intend to apply for an H-1B visa (see below).

The definitive source of information on USMLE exams is the *USMLE Bulletin of Information*, which can found on the USMLE Web site.

TABLE 5-3. **2004 Pass Rates for First-Time USMLE Test Takers**

	U.S. Students (%)	IMGs (%)
Step 1	91	67
Step 2 CK	92	79

The ECFMG Certificate

If you are an IMG, the ECFMG will serve as the rough equivalent of your dean's office in the matching process. ECFMG certification can be a tedious process, but it is essential if you are to be considered by U.S. residencies. Indeed, according to U.S. legal statutes, IMGs who do not have an ECFMG certificate are "invisible" to U.S. residency programs. In addition to passing the required exams, applicants for ECFMG certification must meet certain medical education credential requirements. All IMGs must have had at least four credit years (academic years for which credit has been given toward completion of the medical curriculum) in attendance at a medical school that is listed in the International Medical Education Directory (IMED) on the ECFMG Web site. The physician's graduation year must be included in the medical school's IMED listing.

Additionally, ECFMG requires copies of your medical education credentials, which are verified by the appropriate officials at your medical school. If you have already graduated from medical school when you submit your first application to ECFMG, you must include copies of your medical diploma and a recent photograph with your application. If you are still a student, you must send the copies of your diploma and your photograph as soon as you graduate. You must also provide an English translation if the document you provide is not in English. When ECFMG sends your medical diploma to your medical school for verification, ECFMG will request the medical school to include your final medical school transcript when the school returns the verification of your medical diploma to ECFMG. ECFMG will notify you in writing when it sends your credentials for verification and when it receives verification of your credentials from your medical school.

Be sure to stay on top of the credentialing process.

The Match

See Chapter 1 for general information about the Match.

The National Resident Matching Program (NRMP) Web site has an "Applicant User Guide," which contains specific information for IMGs. IMGs need to fulfill all requirements by September in order to have complete certification prior to submission of the Rank Order Lists (ROL) in mid-January. If you have not passed the USMLE by September, you may not be able to enroll in the NRMP. You may, however, apply for residency positions outside of the Match.

While U.S. medical graduates apply to 8 to 12 programs, IMGs should submit applications to a minimum of 20 to 30 programs, consisting of both teaching and community hospitals. Applications should be sent in as early as possible. While you are waiting, you can begin to research your visa options and even get started on some of the paperwork for medical licensure in the state(s) where you hope to match. On Match Day, if all has gone well, you will know where you are going and can begin to work on your visa.

ERAS

The Electronic Residency Application Service, or ERAS, has almost universally replaced the paper applications of old, transmitting residency applications and credentials via the Internet. It is important to note that some programs and specialties including neurosurgery and ophthalmology still require paper applications. ERAS is available to all U.S. medical graduates as well as those outside the United States and Canada through ECFMG. More information on the ERAS application can be found in Chapter 7.

IMGs are advised to apply to a broad range of programs, as the climate for acceptance can fluctuate from year to year. IMGs should also note that their personal statements will be closely scrutinized for their use and mastery of the English language. Therefore, pay close attention to your personal statement and have it read by a native English speaker. When it comes to proofreading your personal statement, remember that more reviewers looking for mistakes will help you avoid more errors.

Apply to a wide range of

programs to cover your bases.

Interviews

If all has gone well thus far, you will be invited to interview at a subset of the programs to which you applied. You will interview along with U.S. medical graduates on predetermined days and should follow the advice presented in Chapter 11 of this book. There are, however, some additional points that should be mentioned.

- You should get a feel for each program's overall approach to IMGs on the day of your interview. Are there many IMGs at the program, or have there been at least a few in the past?
- Other IMGs are excellent resources from whom you can glean valuable information about immigration issues as well as an idea of the level of support the program provides to IMGs.

The interview is a good time

to get a feeling for how

IMG-friendly a program is.

Keep in mind that a positive experience with an IMG from your medical school in the past may open doors for you in that program.

In addition to the interview tips presented in Chapter 11, consider the following advice:

- Describe your school in the most positive of terms. U.S. program directors and interviewers are not necessarily biased against foreign medical schools, but they are wary of unknown entities.
- If you portray your school in a positive light, it is more likely to be perceived that way.
- It may be prudent to save questions about visas for other residents and program administrators, as program directors may not know this information.
- Keep the discussion on medicine and training, since these are universal goals of residents, applicants, and program directors.
- The goal of your interview should be to convince your interviewer that due to your shared interest in medicine, you both have more in common than he or she may think, even if you are the only IMG the program has ever interviewed.

MAXIMIZING YOUR CHANCES

As an IMG you may face disadvantages when applying to programs at top-tier institutions, such as teaching hospitals affiliated with renowned universities and research centers. In some cases, IMGs will not even be considered for an interview simply because there are too many qualified U.S. graduates from the university's own medical school and other U.S. schools. However, that is not the end of the road for the IMG, because there is a subset of IMGs who continue to match every year at competitive institutions. The following are some ways to maximize your chances as an IMG.

Doing Research

Explore all possible options, beginning with research positions, fellowships, and even research assistantships.

IMGs who prepare well continue to match at competitive programs every year.

- Ironically, most of the big research universities and hospitals usually have multiple opportunities for research-based positions that are simply unfilled.
- These positions may not pay that well or may be unfilled because there are no U.S. medical graduates willing to take up a one- to two-year research fellowship.
- In addition, these very programs also almost always have a research director's office or dean for research. This office can provide the IMG with a very useful list of potential job openings, often with visa support for the right candidate.

The ideal research position is within the department in which the candidates wishes to do a residency. For example, surgical residencies are very competitive; however, over the last few years some IMGs have matched in orthopedics, plastics, and general surgery. They may have started as research fellows, completed one to three years of research, and proved themselves as viable applicants. The goal is to get some recognition through research. Once your name is recognizable via presentations, papers, and publications, program directors might be more willing to rank you favorably.

U.S. research experience will put the IMG ahead of the pack.

Contrary to popular belief, large research-based university centers actually are more open to IMGs since they want to have an international feel—but the IMG has to be known to the program director, faculty, and residents. Working at a well-known research institution increases your chances of being called for interviews by other teaching hospitals. This experience will also give you the opportunity to generate letters of recommendation from U.S. teaching faculty.

It helps if the IMG has had interaction with the program director, faculty, and residents.

Some positions that are open at university hospitals may not be salaried for the first year but provide a stipend for future years. While this may seem unattractive, IMGs who have taken this approach have had good results. Program directors may think highly of applicants who prove their mettle through determination in the face of hardship. In addition, it demonstrates an applicant's ability to work on research projects both independently and as part of a team.

Obtaining an Advanced Degree

Getting advanced degrees in the United States can be a major boost toward getting interviews at desirable programs. The IMG will stand out because of the additional skills, research, and maturity acquired during the program for an MPH or MS degree—attributes that teaching/university programs find attractive. While working toward the advanced degree, it also does no harm for the IMG to try to get more clinical exposure, either through electives and attachments or more informally through clinical conferencing, morning reports, journal clubs, and didactic sessions with the residents of the program.

Given the trend of USMGs earning intercalated degrees, such as an MBA or PhD, during medical school or even residency, an IMG with an advanced degree is all the more competitive. The disadvantage with this strategy is that it is a considerable time commitment and can be a financial burden.

Doing NIH-Funded Research

Although this seems difficult, there are numerous such jobs available at major teaching hospitals. Many principal investigators (PIs) find it difficult to find good research staff once they have managed to get funding from the NIH. An IMG often suits these positions very well because the PI can hire a capable, dedicated MD who can communicate well in medical English. The benefit to you is that any publications resulting from this kind of endeavor greatly increase your chances of matching.

Presenting Research Work for Awards

Often, there are opportunities for presenting research work for an award, however small. Many IMG recipients of research awards have matched at very high-caliber programs. Other IMG applicants started in research and ended up excelling and actually benefiting from their own grants. While their numbers are small, these IMGs almost always can match at a residency of their choice.

Even though most IMGs apply to and match at community hospitals, trying for a position at a university teaching hospital is worthwhile, especially if the IMG has done some research or electives or has written some papers. It is important to remember that differences exist between teaching and community hospitals, although both focus on providing excellent patient care.

Overall, an IMG who is very motivated will typically have more success than one who is content to just apply and wait for interviews. The IMG applicant who is willing to sacrifice one to two years doing research may find that time was well spent, since it led to greater recognition and a match at a good university hospital.

IMMIGRATION

For detailed current immigration information, please visit the U.S. State Department Web site (http://travel.state.gov/visa/).

To attend interviews, IMGs must enter the United States. This can be accomplished with the use of a visitor B-1/B-2 visa. These give you ample time (two to six months) to complete interviews. Once it comes time to start a residency, however, things get a bit more complicated.

As an IMG, you need a visa to work or train in the United States unless you are a U.S. citizen or a permanent resident. Two types of visas enable you to accept a residency appointment in the United States: J-1 and H-1B. Most sponsoring residency programs (SRPs) prefer a J-1 visa. Above all, this is because SRPs are authorized by the Department of Homeland Security (DHS) to issue a Form DS-2019 directly to an IMG. By contrast, SRPs must complete considerable paperwork, including an application to the Immigration and Labor Department, to apply to the DHS for an H-1B visa on behalf of an IMG.

The J-1 Visa

This is a nonimmigrant visa. Key features of this visa include:

- The J1 visa is one of the most restrictive and inflexible visas on which to come to the United States.
- Also known as the Exchange Visitor Program, the J-1 visa was introduced to give IMGs in diverse specialties the chance to use the training experience obtained in the United States in their respective home countries and improve conditions there.
- To enable an SRP to issue a DS-2019, you must obtain a certificate from the ECFMG indicating that you are eligible to participate in a residency program in the United States. First, however, you must have the Ministry of Health in your country to issue a statement indicating that your country needs physicians with the skills you propose to acquire from a U.S. residency program. This statement, which must bear the seal of your country's government and must be signed by a duly designated government official, is intended to satisfy the U.S. Secretary of Health and Human Services (HHS) that there is such a need.

J-1 visas can be very restrictive and inflexible.

The Health Ministry in your country should send this statement to the ECFMG. To find out if the government of your country will issue such a statement, you will likely need to contact the Ministry of Health, which, in many countries, maintains a list of medical specialties in which there is a need for further training abroad. A word of caution: if you are applying for a residency in internal medicine and internists are not in short supply in your country, it may help to indicate an intention to pursue a subspecialty after completing your residency training.

The text of your statement of need should read as follows:

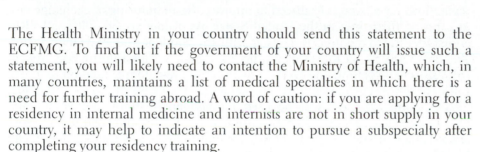

> Name of applicant for visa: _____. There currently exists in _____ (your country) a need for qualified medical practitioners in the specialty of _____. (Name of applicant for visa) has filed a written assurance with the government of this country that he/she will return to _____ (your country) upon completion of training in the United States and intends to enter the practice of medicine in the specialty for which training is being sought.
>
> Stamp (or seal and signature) of issuing official of named country.
>
> Dated _____

To facilitate the issuing of such a statement by the Ministry of Health in your country, you should submit a certified copy of the agreement or a contract from your residency in the United States. The agreement or contract must be signed by you and the residency program official responsible for the training. Armed with Form DS-2019, you should then go to the U.S. consulate closest to the residential address indicated in your passport.

Nonimmigrant Intent

J-1 visa applicants must demonstrate to the consulate officer that they have binding ties to a residence in their home country which they have no intention of abandoning, and that they are coming to the United States for a temporary period. As for other nonimmigrant visas, you must prove that you intend to return to your home country. This intent is established in part by demonstrating that you have financial assets and personal ties in your home country. You must also show that all your expenses will be paid. In addition, you may need a certificate of good conduct, which is usually obtained through the medical board in your country.

Usually, after security clearance and authenticating your documents, the U.S. consulate will authorize the visa. Currently, this process can take anywhere between one and six months, depending on your home country. When you enter the United States, be sure to carry *all* your documents, including your Form DS-2019 and the visa letters you initially submitted to the U.S. embassy at home. Sometimes the INS officers at the port of entry will ask to see these despite your having a visa. You are usually admitted to the United States for the length of the J-1 program, designated as "D/S," or duration of status. The duration of your program is indicated on the DS-2019.

In the wake of the terrorist attacks of September 11, 2001, a number of new regulations have been introduced to improve the monitoring of exchange visitors during their time in the United States. As of January 30, 2003, all SRPs and students are required to register with the Student and Exchange Visitor Program (SEVP) via the Student and Exchange Visitor Information System (SEVIS). SEVIS allows the DHS to maintain up-to-date information (e.g., enrollment status, current address) on exchange visitors. As of January 30, 2002, SEVIS Form DS-2019 will be used for visa applications, admission, and change of status. Non-SEVIS forms, such as Form IAP-66, issued before January 30, 2003, are no longer accepted. Procedural details of this legislation can be obtained from your SRP, the international office at your institution, or the DHS Web site.

Duration of participation. The duration of a resident's participation in a program of graduate medical education or training is limited to the time normally required to complete such a program. The authority charged with determining the duration of time required by an individual IMG is the State Department. The maximum amount of time for participation in a training program is ordinarily limited to seven years unless the IMG has demonstrated to the satisfaction of the ECFMG and the U.S. State Department that his or her home country has an exceptional need for the specialty in which he or she will receive further training. An extension of stay may be granted in the event that an IMG needs to repeat a year of clinical medical training or needs time for training or education to take an exam required for board certification. After the seven years have elapsed, the IMG is required by law to either travel back to his/her home country or pursue a waiver of this requirement. The waiver process can take up to or more than a year, so if you intend to apply for one, start early. More details are provided in the "J-1 Waiver" section below. Please refer to the visa section of the State Department's Web site (http://travel.state.gov/visa/).

Requirements after entry into the United States. Each year, all IMGs participating in a residency program on a J-1 visa must furnish the attorney general of the United States with an affidavit (Form I-644) attesting that they are in good standing in the program of graduate medical education or training in which they are participating and that they will return to their home country upon completion of the education or training for which they came to the United States.

Allow adequate time for security and immigration clearances when applying for visas.

Restrictions under the J-1 visa. No later than two years after the date of entry into the United States, an IMG participating in a residency program on a J-1 visa is allowed one opportunity to change his or her designated program of graduate medical education or training if his or her director approves that change. The J-1 visa also includes a condition called the "two-year foreign residence requirement." The law requires that a J-1 visa holder, upon completion of the training program, leave the United States and reside in his or her home country for a period of at least two years. Currently, there is pressure from the American Medical Association to extend this period to five years. An IMG on a J-1 visa is ordinarily not allowed to change from J-1 to most other types of visas or (in most cases) to change from J-1 to permanent residence while in the United States until he or she has fulfilled the "foreign residence requirement." The purpose of the foreign residence requirement is to ensure that an IMG uses the training he or she obtained in the United States for the benefit of his or her home country.

J-2 visas/family members. The spouse and children (minors only) of participants in exchange programs may apply for J-2 dependent visas to accompany and join the IMG on the J-1 visa. They must demonstrate that they will have sufficient financial resources to cover all expenses while in the United States. Dependents may apply to the U.S. Citizenship and Immigration Services (USCIS, formerly the Immigration and Naturalization Service) for authorization to accept employment in the United States.

Some individuals may apply for a waiver of the two-year foreign residency requirement. There are five grounds for which the U.S. government may waive the two-year foreign residence requirement:

- If you as an IMG can prove that returning to your country would result in "exceptional hardship" to you or to members of your immediate family who are U.S. citizens or permanent residents;
- If you as an IMG can demonstrate a "well-founded fear of persecution" due to race, religion, or political opinions if forced to return to your country;
- If you obtain a "no objection" statement from your government;
- If you are sponsored by an "interested governmental agency"; or
- If you are sponsored by a designated state Department of Health in the United States.

By far the most commonly used reason and possibly the least rejected application is the "interested governmental agency" sponsoring the IMG.

Applying for a J-1 visa waiver. IMGs who have sought a waiver on the basis of the last two alternatives have found it beneficial to approach the following potentially "interested government agencies":

1. **The Department of Health and Human Services.** As of 2003, HHS has expanded its role in reviewing J-1 waiver applications. HHS's considerations for a waiver have classically been as follows:

   - The program or activity in which the IMG is engaged is "of high priority and of national or international significance in an area of interest" to HHS;
   - The IMG must be an "integral" part of the program or activity "so that the loss of his/her services would necessitate discontinuance of the program or a major phase of it"; and

- The IMG "must possess outstanding qualifications, training, and experience well beyond the usually expected accomplishments at the graduate, postgraduate, and residency levels and must clearly demonstrate the capability to make original and significant contributions to the program."

Under these criteria, HHS waivers are granted to physicians working in high-level biomedical research.

New rules will also allow HHS to review J-1 waiver applications from community health centers, rural hospitals, and other health care providers. In the past, the U.S. Department of Agriculture (USDA) served as the interested federal government agency that reviewed waiver applications to allow foreign doctors to serve in rural underserved communities outside Appalachia, while the Appalachian Regional Commission (ARC) played that role for Appalachian communities. The USDA is no longer handling applications for J-1 waivers. As such, HHS will now review waiver applications for primary care practitioners and psychiatrists who have completed residency training within one year of application to practice in designated Health Professional Shortage Areas (HPSAs), Medically Underserved Areas and Populations (MUA/Ps), and Mental Health Professional Shortage Areas (MHPSAs). HHS waiver applications should be mailed to:

> Executive Secretary
> Exchange Visitor Waiver Review Board
> Room 639-H, Hubert H. Humphrey Building
> Department of Health and Human Services
> 200 Independence Avenue, S.W.
> Washington, D.C. 20201
> Phone (202) 690-6174; fax (202) 690-7127

2. **Veterans Affairs.** With more than 170 health care facilities located in various parts of the United States, the VA is a major employer of physicians in this country. In addition, many VA hospitals are affiliated with university medical centers. The VA sponsors IMGs working in research, patient care (regardless of specialty), and teaching.

The waiver applicant may engage in teaching and research in conjunction with clinical duties. The VA's latest guidelines (issued on June 22, 1994) provide that it will act as an interested government agency only when the loss of the IMG's services would necessitate the discontinuance of a program or a major phase of it and when recruitment efforts have failed to locate a U.S. physician to fill the position.

The procedure for obtaining a VA sponsorship for a J-1 waiver is as follows:

- The IMG should deal directly with the Human Resources Department at the local VA facility; and
- The facility must request that the VA's chief medical director sponsor the IMG for a waiver.

The waiver request should include the following documentation:

- A letter from the director of the local facility describing the program, the IMG's immigration status, the health care needs of the facility, and the facility's recruitment efforts;
- Recruitment efforts, including copies of all job advertisements run within the preceding year; and
- Copies of the IMG's licenses, test results, board certifications, SEVIS

DS-2019 forms, etc. The VA contact person in Washington, D.C., should be contacted by the local medical facility rather than by IMGs or their attorneys.

3. **The Appalachian Regional Commission.** The ARC sponsors physicians in certain places in the eastern and southern United States, namely, in Alabama, Georgia, Kentucky, Maryland, Mississippi, New York, North Carolina, Ohio, Pennsylvania, South Carolina, Tennessee, Virginia, and West Virginia. Since 1992, the ARC has sponsored approximately 200 primary care IMGs annually in counties within its jurisdiction that have been designated as HPSAs by HHS. The ARC requires that waiver requests initially be submitted to the ARC contact person in the state of intended employment. Contact information for each state can be found on the ARC Web site (www.arc.gov). If the state concurs, a letter from the state's governor recommending the waiver must be addressed to Anne B. Pope, the new federal co-chairperson of the ARC. The waiver request should include the following documents:

- A letter from the facility to Executive Secretary, Exchange Visitor Waiver Review Board stating the proposed dates of employment, the IMG's medical specialty, the address of the practice location, an assertion that the IMG will practice primary care for at least 40 hours per week in the HPSA, and details as to why the facility needs the services of the IMG;
- A J-1 Visa Data Sheet;
- The ARC federal co-chairperson's J-1 Visa Waiver Policy and the J-1 Visa Waiver Policy Affidavit and Agreement with the notarized signature of the IMG;
- A contract of at least three years' duration;
- Evidence of the IMG's qualifications, including a résumé, medical diplomas and licenses, and IAP-66 or SEVIS DS-2019 forms; and
- Evidence of unsuccessful attempts to recruit qualified U.S. physicians within the preceding six months. Copies of advertisements, copies of résumés received, and reasons for rejection must also be included.

The ARC will not sponsor IMGs who have been out of status for six months or longer. Requests for ARC waivers are then processed in Washington, D.C. (ARC, 1666 Connecticut Avenue, N.W., Washington, D.C. 20009).

The ARC is usually able to forward a letter confirming that a waiver has been recommended to the United States Information Agency (USIA) to the requesting facility or attorney within 30 days of the request.

4. **The Department of Agriculture.** At the time of publication, the USDA is no longer sponsoring J-1 waivers. The scope of the HHS J-1 waiver program has been expanded to fill the gap.

5. **State Departments of Public Health.** There is no application form for a state-sponsored J-1 waiver. However, USIA regulations specify that an application must include the following documents:

- A letter from the state Department of Public Health identifying the physician and specifying that it would be in the public interest to grant him or her a J-1 waiver;
- An employment contract that is valid for a minimum of three years and that states the name and address of the facility that will employ the physician and the geographic areas in which he or she will practice medicine;

- Evidence that these geographic areas are located within HPSAs;
- A statement by the physician agreeing to the contractual requirements;
- Copies of all SEVIS DS-2019 forms; and
- A completed USIA Data Sheet.

Applications are numbered in the order in which they are received, since only 30 physicians per year may be granted waivers in a particular state under the Conrad State 30 program. Individual states may choose to participate or not to participate in this program. At the time of publication, nonparticipating states included Idaho, Oklahoma, and Wyoming, while Texas had suspended its J-1 waiver program pending new legislation.

The H-1B Visa

Since 1991, the law has allowed medical residency programs to sponsor foreign-born medical residents for H-1B visas. There are no restrictions to changing the H-1B visa to any other kind of visa, including permanent resident status (green card), through employer sponsorship or through close relatives who are U.S. citizens or permanent residents. The overall ceiling for the number of H-1B visas issued to professionals in all categories was increased to 195,000 for the years 2002–2003. This ceiling is scheduled to revert to 65,000 visas in 2004–2005. It is advisable for residents to apply for H-1B visas as soon as possible in the official year (beginning October 1) when the new quota officially opens up. According to the Web site www.immihelp.com, the following beneficiaries of approved H-1B petitions are exempt from the H-1B annual cap:

- Beneficiaries who are in J-1 nonimmigrant status in order to receive graduate medical education or training, and who have obtained a waiver of the two-year home residency requirement.
- Beneficiaries who are employed at, or who have received an offer of employment from, an institution of higher education or a related or affiliated nonprofit entity.
- Beneficiaries who are employed by, or who have received an offer of employment from, a nonprofit research organization.
- Beneficiaries who are employed by, or who have received an offer of employment from, a governmental research organization.
- Beneficiaries who are currently maintaining, or who have held within the last six years, H-1B status, and are ineligible for another full six-year stay as an H-1B.
- Beneficiaries who have been counted once toward the numerical limit and are the beneficiary of multiple petitions.

H-1B visas are intended for "professionals" in a "specialty occupation." This means that an IMG intending to pursue a residency program in the United States with an H-1B visa needs to clear all three USMLE Steps before becoming eligible for the H-1B. The ECFMG administers Steps 1 and 2, whereas Step 3 is conducted by the individual states. Most states will not allow medical residents to take USMLE Step 3 until they have completed the first year of their residency programs. However, there are 11 states that permit persons to take USMLE Step 3 prior to entering a residency program: Connecticut, Arkansas, California, Florida, Louisiana, Maryland, Nevada, New York, Texas, Virginia, and West Virginia. IMGs interested in being sponsored for H-1B status must travel to one of these states to take and pass USMLE Step 3 before they may be sponsored for an H-1B visa.

You will need to contact the Federation of State Medical Boards (FSMB) or the medical board of the state where you intend to take the Step 3 for additional details.

H-1B Application

An application for an H-1B visa is filed not by the IMG but rather by his or her employment sponsor—in your case, by the residency program in the United States. If an SRP is willing to do so, you will be told about it at the time of your interview for the residency program. If an SRP is unwilling to file for an H-1B visa because of attorney costs, you could suggest that you would be willing to bear the burden of such costs. The entire process of getting an H-1B visa can take anywhere from 10 to 20 weeks.

More IMGs are obtaining the H-1B visa since it is less restrictive.

The physician may not commence employment in the United States until the petition is approved and the physician has either H-1B status or has obtained an H-1B visa and entered the United States. With H-4 visas, a spouse and unmarried children under 21 years old can accompany an H-1B physician and may attend school in the United States, but they cannot work. The initial duration of an H-1B petition is three years, with one additional three-year extension of stay possible. Generally, after six years have elapsed, the physician must either have permanent residence status or depart the United States.

The events of September 11 have led to dramatic changes for all immigrants seeking to enter the United States. The information outlined above as well as in the rest of this book should give you a deeper understanding of the process of matching in the United States as an IMG. That said, just as medicine always changes, so too do procedures for immigration. Do not allow lack of information to prevent your residency dreams from coming true!

IMG RESOURCES

- For information on the ECFMG and on Steps 1 and 2 of the USMLE, including application forms, contact:

  Educational Commission for Foreign Medical Graduates
  3624 Market Street
  Philadelphia, PA 19104-2685
  (215) 386-5900
  www.ecfmg.org

- For general information regarding the USMLE, contact:

  USMLE Secretariat
  3750 Market Street
  Philadelphia, PA 19104-3190
  (215) 590-9600
  www.usmle.org

- For general information on medical licensure and Step 3 of the USMLE, contact:

  Federation of State Medical Boards
  P.O. Box 619850
  Dallas, TX 75261-9850
  (817) 868-4000
  Fax: (817) 868-4099
  www.fsmb.org

- For detailed information on the USMLE Step 3 and specific licensure issues, contact the state Board of Medical Examiners in the state in which you wish to practice.
- For further information on the NRMP or to request an NRMP application, contact:

National Resident Matching Program
2450 N Street, N.W.
Washington, D.C. 20037-1127
(202) 828-0566
www.nrmp.org

Please include your USMLE/ECFMG identification number on all correspondence.

- For information on visas and immigration services, contact:

Bureau of Citizenship and Immigration Services
425 I Street, N.W.
Washington, D.C. 20536
(800) 375-5283
www.immigration.gov

American Immigration Lawyers Association
www.aila.org
(800) 982-2839

- For IMG resources offered by the American Medical Association, contact:

American Medical Association
Department of IMG Services
515 N. State Street
Chicago, IL 60610
(312) 464-5728
www.ama-assn.org/go/imgs

- For additional information about the Exchange Visitor Sponsorship Program for foreign national physicians sponsored by the ECFMG, contact:

ECFMG Exchange Visitor Sponsorship Program
P.O. Box 41673
Philadelphia, PA 19101-1673
(215) 662-1445
Fax: (215) 386-9766

- For further information on the Electronic Residency Application Service (ERAS), contact:

ECFMG/ERAS Program
P.O. Box 13467
Philadelphia, PA 19101-3467
(215) 386-5900
Fax: (215) 222-5641
www.aamc.org/audienceeras.htm

- For information on Health Professional Shortage Areas (HPSA), contact:

Bureau of Primary Health Care
Division of Shortage Designation
4350 East-West Highway
Bethesda, MD 20814
(301) 594-0816

Online Database of HPSAs:
http://bphc.hrsa.gov/

- For information on ARC, contact:

Appalachian Regional Commission
1666 Connecticut Avenue, NW
Washington, D.C. 20235
(202) 884-7700
www.arc.gov

- For information on the VA, contact:

U.S. Department of Veterans Affairs
810 Vermont Avenue, NW
Washington, D.C. 20420
(800) 827-1000
www.va.gov

References

Garibaldi RA, Subhiyah R, Moore ME, Waxman H. The in-training examination in internal medicine: an analysis of resident perfomance over time. *Ann Intern Med* 137(6):505–510, 2002.

Moore RA, Rhodenbaugh EJ: The unkindest cut of all: are IMGS subjected to discrimination by general surgery residency programs? *Curr Surg* 59(2):228–236, 2002.

National Resident Matching Program 2005 Match Data, www.nrmp.org/res_match/tables/-table2_05.pdf.

Norcini JJ, Boulet JR, Whelan GP, McKinley DW. Specialty Board certification among U.S. citizen and non-U.S. citizen graduates of international medical schools. *Acad Med* 80(10 Suppl):S42–45, 2005.

Polsky D, Kletke PR, Wozniak GD, Escarce JJ. Initial practice locations of IMGs. *Health Serv Res* 37(4):907–928, 2002.

Whelan GP, Gary NE, Kostis J, Boulet JR, Hallock JA. The changing pool of international medical graduates seeking certification training in U.S. graduate medical education programs. *JAMA* 288(9):1079–1084, 2002.

NOTES

CHAPTER 6

Getting Residency Information and Applications

A wealth of information is at your fingertips. Begin your search early and remember to organize!

Throughout the application season, you will be gathering and reviewing a lot of information. This information will include the specifics of particular residency programs, housing, cost of living, benefits, and information about the interview itself. As you can imagine, the details can become overwhelming! Many students realize far too late that they have not organized the information appropriately. A lack of preparation could mean missed interviews, overlooked details, and forgotten follow-up letters are not sent, with the obvious negative effects on Match Day.

How can you prevent this from happening to you? It's simple: organize early and often! At the end of your third year, purchase a stack of manila folders or expanding folders so that you can create a file system. As you begin to research programs, place all materials concerning each program in a separate respective folder. As you receive interview invitations, include these in the folders, along with interview confirmations, travel plans, and notes created after the interview. If you lose interest in a program, simply toss the entire folder! For those who prefer an electronic filing system (i.e., on a computer or PDA), remember to keep a paper backup.

Be sure to keep copies of interview confirmations! Secretaries can be busy, and you would hate to get lost in the shuffle.

An "interview calendar" should also be set up at this time. You should use the table on the inside front cover to roughly fill in this calendar. Then, as you set up specific interview dates, you can use the calendar to consolidate dates.

This basic preemptive organization process will serve you well. Once you have a place for everything, you can start putting everything in its place. You can now begin the search for the residency of your dreams.

Before you start the application process, you will need to acquire enough information about available residency programs to make a list of programs that fit your needs. Fortunately, there is no scarcity of data available on training programs (see Table 6-1). In fact, you will have to be selective and efficient in your information gathering. Career advisers, for example, can provide a broad perspective on a number of programs, including clinical training and research. On the other hand, junior faculty, fellows, and house staff can draw from their own residency experience to give you the nitty-gritty about training at specific programs. However, there is no one source that will tell you everything you need to know as it relates to your goals. Therefore, use enough sources to get the necessary information.

Resources abound at your medical school. Use them!

Career Adviser/Mentor

Your career adviser/mentor should be aware of your personal and professional goals, and therefore be able to help identify programs that will best fit your needs. In addition, your adviser often can provide information regarding the "personality" of various programs. For instance, he or she may be able to identify the current department chair, academic and clinical foci, and overall reputation of the research that is conducted at a particular institution. He or she may also be aware of recent graduates from your medical school who are currently training at a given institution. If so, obtain your adviser's contact information and take advantage of the knowledge and insight he or she may have

112

TABLE 6-1. Information Resources for Residency Programs

SOURCE	CONTRIBUTION
Career adviser (department chairperson, clinical faculty)	To identify appropriate programs to apply to and inform you of the current status of each.
Dean of students	To help you choose between specialties, pick an adviser, and assess overall competitiveness.
Faculty and house staff	To provide perspective on training and residency life.
Fourth-year medical students	To summarize what's hot/what's not: tips and warnings for prospects in your specialty.
AMA Fellowship and Residency Electronic Interactive Database (AMA-FREIDA) Web site (www.ama-assn.org/ama/pub/category/2997.htm)	To provide current contact information for your target programs as well as detailed statistics.
Graduate Medical Education Directory (the "Green Book")	To provide contacts for residency programs. Next best thing to FREIDA.
NRMP Program Results: Listing of Filled and Unfilled Programs (available on the NRMP Web site at www.nrmp.org)	To list the programs that did not fill all their spots in the previous Match.
Transitional Year Program Directory (the "Purple Book")	To give detailed listings of transitional-year programs.
Directories published by some specialties	To supplement or update information in FREIDA.
San Francisco Matching Program Web site (www.sfmatch.org)	To obtain detailed information on the match process for neurology, neurosurgery, and ophthalmology programs.
American Urological Association (AUA) Web site (www.auanet.org)	To obtain detailed information on the match process for urology residency programs.

into a specific program. If this is not the case, be proactive and request copies of Match results from the last three graduating classes from your medical school and make phone calls on your own.

Dean of Students

It is surprising how many students pass up the opportunity to make an appointment with the dean of students, perhaps out of fear that the dean is "too busy" to speak with them or is absorbed with weightier matters. Don't hesitate to schedule an appointment, as this faculty member can be an excellent source of information, advice, and advocacy. Even a brief meeting with your dean can give you inside information about the workings of the Match at your

The dean of students is an often overlooked resource.

school, advance word on how and when the dean's letter will be written, an early assessment of your academic progress as it might influence your specialty and program choice, and suggestions about who the "hot" advisers are. It is never too early to get some hints about strategies, both academic and personal. Don't forget, many deans have gone through this process themselves, often in the not-too-distant past.

Faculty and House Staff

Faculty in your desired specialty whom you meet on your junior and senior clerkships can complement information your career adviser provides. You should therefore talk to as many of these people as possible and make an effort to understand their perspectives (e.g., geographic, academic versus clinical). Senior residents can share their sense of the job market as well as their own job-hunting experiences. Junior faculty and fellows can shed light on the residency programs that trained them. Especially valuable in this regard are junior faculty who trained elsewhere, as these individuals have a recent yet mature perspective on how a particular training program differs from others—or at least how that program differs from the one at your institution. Junior faculty are often enthusiastic about getting involved with students.

To a certain extent, the same holds true of house staff, who can readily provide information on programs they knew as medical students. Bear in mind, however, that the perspective of house staff is limited to their own program and does not necessarily apply to any others. House staff may also lack the "big picture," just as you do. Interns in their third month of residency, as sleep-deprived and cranky as they tend to be, are unlikely to shed many pearls of wisdom about your future.

Senior Medical Students

Inasmuch as they have survived their interviews and Match Day, graduating seniors are your best bet for practical application and interviewing tips. Debriefing some of these survivors will give you an additional "feel" for the application process and alert you to potential trouble spots. Most medical schools organize question-and-answer sessions with graduating seniors. Remember, though, that while seniors have considerable "trench" experience, their perspectives are understandably limited when it comes to what programs might be best for you.

Outside Faculty

If your medical school is affiliated with a VA, county, or private hospital, keep the faculty at these institutions in mind as potential sources of advice. Although medical students have historically underutilized such faculty members, many have considerable insight into aspects of medical training that their more academic colleagues in the Ivory Tower lack. For example, they may know of special loan repayment programs offered to VA residents, may be aware of the "job track" at HMOs such as Kaiser Permanente, and may be adept at comparing one county facility with another in terms of training.

Fellows from other institutions can provide valuable comparisons between programs.

Fellowship and Residency Electronic Interactive Database (FREIDA)

FREIDA (www.ama-assn.org/ama/pub/category/2997.htm) is an annually updated, PC-based database of residency programs that is produced by the American Medical Association (AMA). If you use only one resource to gather initial information on residency programs, this should be it. FREIDA contains information on approximately 7500 graduate medical programs and combined programs that are accredited by the Accreditation Council for Graduate Medical Education (ACGME). It is very easy to use and has supplanted the *Graduate Medical Education Directory* (aka the "Green Book") as the most popular source on residency programs. The data within it are derived from the AMA Annual Survey of Graduate Medical Education Programs. These surveys are filled out in the fall and the data are entered in both October and February. Programs can change some of the basic information throughout the year.

Accessed through the Internet, FREIDA can search for programs by specialty, region or state, and optional criteria, such as program size, preliminary positions available, and many more, dividing an overwhelming amount of information on each program into eight manageable categories (see Table 6-2). Included in each program's basic information are the name, address, phone number, and e-mail address of the program director and contact person, and the program's Web site address, all of which can help students obtain answers to questions not answered by FREIDA. Each program has a ten-digit identifying number that will be listed in the "Search Results" page as well as under the program's basic information. Writing down these numbers will enable you to bypass the search engine and go directly to that specific program's information in the future.

FREIDA has two other categories. The category of "Specialty Statistics" provides general information on specialties and subspecialties, such as work hours, work environment, and average compensation. "Physician Workforce Information" provides statistics given by residents and practicing physicians on finding employment, workplace environment, job satisfaction, and the like. There are, however, a few things you should remember about FREIDA. First, the information is sometimes incomplete or outdated. Double check information from FREIDA with information provided on individual program Web sites or the residency program coordinator. Second, all information is provided by the programs themselves, and none of it is verified. Sometimes program directors choose not to answer certain questions that they feel are irrelevant or embarrassing. Other programs do not fill out questionnaires at all and are listed only by name. Finally, keep in mind that as a self-reporting database, FREIDA does not evaluate or compare programs objectively.

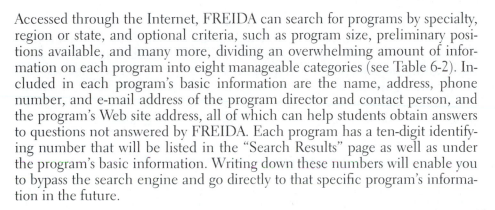

TABLE 6-2.
Information in FREIDA

General program information
Educational environment
Work environment
Compensation and benefits
Clinical environment
Patient population
Medical benefits/institution features
Specialties in institution

Graduate Medical Education Directory: The "Green Book"

The *Graduate Medical Education Directory* is an annually updated catalog of all training programs recognized by the ACGME. Despite its heft, the directory has very little information for each program other than the contact address and telephone number (see Table 6-3).

The Green Book can be obtained at your office of student affairs or medical library. You can order your own copy online at www.ama-assn.org or call toll free (800) 621-8335.

TABLE 6-3. Information in "Green Book" Program Listing

Program director's name, address, telephone number
Sponsoring institution
Other institutions with a major role in training
Number of training years
Total number of positions in program
Program ID number

If you are an IMG with no convenient access to FREIDA, you should probably purchase your own copy of the Green Book. Although the program information contained in it is not as extensive as that in FREIDA, the Green Book does feature *some* facts that FREIDA does not cover. These include visa and certification guidelines for foreign-born medical graduates seeking graduate medical education in the United States; detailed ACGME requirements for program accreditation by specialty; and state licensure requirements.

Transitional Year Program Directory: The "Purple Book"

The Purple Book lists most transitional-year programs and includes contact information as well as data on required and elective rotations, call schedule, and the like. Given that much of the same information is available in FREIDA, you should use the Purple Book as a secondary resource. It should be available at your office of student affairs and is also available over the Internet (www.ahme.org). A copy can be ordered by calling or writing:

> Association for Hospital Medical Education (AHME)
> 419 Beulah Road
> Pittsburgh, PA 15235
> (412) 244-9302

NRMP Program Results: Listing of Filled and Unfilled Programs

As described in Chapter 1, the NRMP Program Results lists all programs that did not fill their spots in the NRMP Match. If you are a weak candidate in a strong field, you might want to take a closer look at these programs. If this publication is not available at your student affairs office, you can order it for $45 by calling or writing:

> Attention: Membership and Publication Orders
> National Resident Matching Program
> 2450 N Street, N.W.
> Washington, D.C. 20037-1127
> (202) 828-0416

Specialty-Specific Directories

Several specialty organization Web sites maintain directories of training programs with contact information. In addition, a handful of directories (including those from family practice, internal medicine, psychiatry, physical medicine and rehabilitation, and preventive medicine) rival or surpass FREIDA in terms of comprehensiveness and appropriateness of information. Many of these directories maintain board pass rates for each program. In general, however, the specialty directories are not updated as frequently as FREIDA or the Green Book. See Chapter 4 for a list of specialty organization Web site addresses and contact information.

Early Match Web Sites

For information on neurology, plastic surgery, neurosurgery, and ophthalmology programs, go to the San Francisco Matching Program Web site at www.sf-match.org. Information on urology programs can be found in the "Residency" section at the American Urological Association Web site (www.auanet.org).

HOW MANY PROGRAMS SHOULD I APPLY TO?

Most students want to submit enough applications to yield a healthy number of interviews, which will in turn help ensure a successful match. At the same time, the number of programs you apply to depends on a variety of additional factors, including (1) your competitive standing; (2) the competitiveness of the specialty; (3) the competitiveness of the programs to which you are applying; and (4) whether you're participating in the couples match. Because so many factors figure into this equation, it's best to consult your career adviser or dean to help determine the "right" number for you. If you are even mildly interested in a particular program, however, write or call for an information packet (and an application if it is a non-ERAS [Electronic Residency Application Service] residency program). If you remain unsure, err on the side of submitting too many applications (see Figure 6-1). Don't worry about going overboard at this point, as it is better to decline interview invitations later than to realize that you do not have enough interviews to ensure a good match.

You should also consider the "Rule of Thirds" in your efforts to achieve a balanced set of applications and minimize your chances of not matching. A third of your applications should go to your "dream programs" regardless of their competitiveness. Another third should include desirable programs where you have a solid chance of matching. The last third should consist of acceptable programs that can serve as backups. While this category does not necessitate as many entries as the first two tiers, it is good to have a few programs in the

It is far better to apply to too many programs than to too few.

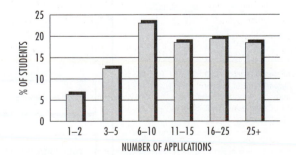

FIGURE 6-1. Number of residency applications made by U.S. fourth-year medical students.

"backup" category. The Rule of Thirds works best in the less competitive specialties. Because of the recent implementation of ERAS and the ease of sending out applications, residency programs are receiving a higher volume of applications in comparison to previous years. See Chapter 4 to find a general prescription for a healthy number of applications in each field.

HOW DO I OBTAIN APPLICATIONS?

The widespread use of ERAS by most specialties has greatly simplified the process of obtaining applications. In fact, for most programs ERAS is the only application you'll need. The application materials are generally available after June 30. Through ERAS, you will complete one common application that can be modified in terms of which letters of recommendation or personal statement you wish to be included for each residency program you apply to.

For those specialties that do not use ERAS, use FREIDA or the Green Book to contact programs for applications. Unfortunately, this is the step that triggers an avalanche of paperwork. To keep yourself sane during this process, **follow two rules from the start.** First, finalize your list of target programs before beginning the application process. Second, try to complete each step of each application at the same time. For example, request all required transcripts in one sitting.

To request applications, purchase prestamped postcards at the post office. If you're using a word processor, it will be worth the effort to create three sets of labels. On the first set, write a brief note requesting information and an application. Type your address on the second set, and enter the name of the program director and the program addresses on the third set. Then, simply attach the three labels to the face of the postcard in the appropriate spots (see Figure 6-2).

You should send for applications and program information **no later than early August.** Allow two to three weeks to receive applications from programs; then

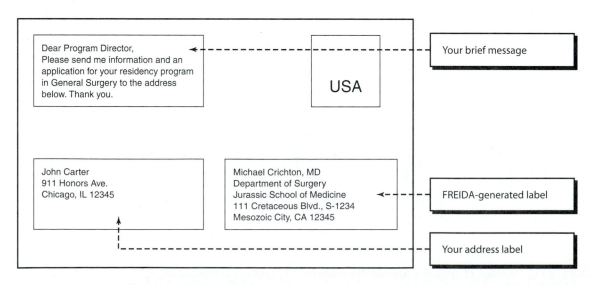

FIGURE 6-2. Sample application request postcard.

follow up with phone calls as needed. If you fall behind on your requests, consider calling all the programs directly for information and applications. It's worth the cost of the phone calls, and you might be able to get answers to some simple questions while you're requesting applications.

WHAT SHOULD I BE LOOKING FOR IN A PROGRAM?

Before you set up your list of programs to apply to, you need to have some idea of your priorities. Although you don't need crystal-ball clarity at this point, you should think through the following issues early in the process, preferably before you start interviewing.

Location

Location is a critical yet highly personal issue. Some candidates are restricted by the employment requirements of their significant other. Other students want to be near family or wish to use residency as an opportunity to establish contacts in the community where they ultimately hope to practice. If you are adventurous and have no serious "attachments," consider programs that will place you on new terrain. Many students who are doing preliminary or transitional PGY-1 years take advantage of the opportunity to experience another city with a limited time commitment. After all, this might be your last chance to do so before marital and family responsibilities catch up with you.

Experience tells us that once students get settled in a city and become accustomed to a particular program, they are often reluctant to leave. They must then scramble during their busy intern year to find a way to stay put. It is important to consider this possibility when applying to programs, even if you initially intend to stay there for just your transitional or preliminary year.

Some locations are incredibly popular, and programs in these areas may be more competitive (see Table 6-4). If there is a particular location that is desirable to you, be sure to apply to a wealth of programs in that region to increase your chances of matching there. Keep in mind that by limiting yourself geographically, you may need to compromise on other program attributes that you are seeking.

Finally, regional variations in style and attitudes can affect residency training. During your interviews, you may detect some regional variations in medical training. The most important thing is to choose the style that best suits you!

TABLE 6-4. Some Application Hot Spots
Boston
Chicago
Hawaii
San Diego
San Francisco
Seattle

Setting

Most applicants' career plans can be categorized as academically oriented, clinically oriented, or both. You want to find a program that fits your preferences. The majority of programs can be classified into the following settings: university, community, urban/county, or health maintenance organization (HMO). Many of these programs run services at more than one hospital, thus offering their residents exposure to multiple settings. It is worth your while to ask about the amount of time you would spend at each hospital.

University. A university medical school affiliation is advantageous for two reasons: (1) medical schools offer teaching opportunities; and (2) the presence of medical students ensures a setting geared toward teaching the residents as well. Teaching conferences are generally of higher quality in university programs than in other settings, although this is not always the case. There are, however, a few drawbacks. For starters, university programs can be more intense, which tends to contribute to a lower level of sociability among the residents. Residents in university programs tend to have greater access to knowledgeable consultants, but some residents complain that because of this wealth of specialists and consultants, they have less autonomy and decision-making responsibility. On one hand, patient populations in a university setting are sometimes not representative of what the resident will encounter in community practice after training. On the other hand, university programs tend to be based in tertiary care centers that give their residents exposure to more unusual or interesting cases.

Community. There is great variability among community programs; however, it is often felt that residents receive a kinder, gentler training in these institutions. In addition, the benefits and salary may also be more generous, and residents are often more relaxed, with less academic pressure and more time for reading. However, some programs may be less academically prestigious, lack formalized educational conferences, and have a large proportion of private patients/attendings. Keep in mind that you may not have the same degree of patient responsibility or diversity of disease experience with less common procedures.

Urban/county. If you really want hands-on experience, city and county hospitals will virtually give you blisters. You can forget academic theorization here; you'll be taught to manage a large patient population consisting primarily of urban poor. Most likely, you will also be heavily involved in the decision-making process and will gain experience with a variety of invasive procedures. Unfortunately, county and city hospital personnel are frequently overworked and underpaid. Moreover, these programs often lack the academic prestige and name recognition of their university equivalents, with notable exceptions such as Massachusetts General Hospital and San Francisco General. In addition, ancillary support tends to be weaker, and formal teaching is often uneven and disorganized.

HMOs. Health maintenance organizations, or HMOs, often have their own hospitals, especially on the West Coast. A number of these hospitals have their own residency programs in some of the larger specialties such as internal medicine. Several other residency programs at academic hospitals have their residents rotate through these HMO hospitals or clinics so that residents have an idea of how these systems work when it comes time for them to apply for positions after residency. HMOs have become a reality in the United States, and they are a viable residency option for many students who like saner hours, appreciate continuity of care, and have an interest in controlling costs in medicine.

Sweeping changes in health care finances make stability a key issue in county and private programs.

Stability

With graduate medical education facing drastic cuts in federal funding, it is important that you determine how financially secure a residency program is. How much of the program's funding comes from federal sources? How well off is the parent hospital or university? County hospitals in several California cities are on the brink of financial collapse; mergers have changed the rotation options of residents in New York and Boston. Hospitals in Denver have closed entirely, leaving residents there jobless. In addition, many teaching hospitals (especially on the East and West Coasts) are now experiencing unprecedented competition from managed care. Does the parent hospital enjoy a robust patient base, or is it floundering in a rising tide of managed care? Although you can do little to change the fiscal policy of a state or the financial pressures motivating a merger, you can take steps to remain aware of these entities and factor them into your ultimate decision.

In addition to financial stability, residencies must be accredited in order to train residents. It is therefore worth your while to see if a program has or recently had any problems with accreditation. Probation is a red flag indicating that something is wrong in the residency, but it may or may not indicate that the problem is being addressed. If your program fails to get accredited after a probation period, you may not be board eligible in the field in which you trained.

Reputation

A program's reputation invariably comes into play if an applicant is considering fellowship training or a career in academic medicine. That reputation, whether deserved or not, can greatly influence your ability to secure competitive fellowships or faculty appointments in the future. If a program is too large, however, prestige doesn't matter; you may still have to sweat to get the strong personal recommendations you need to secure a competitive fellowship. The reality in community practice is that most patients will not know or really care what medical school you graduated from, much less where you trained.

Subspecialty Strengths

If you're considering subspecialty training after residency, you might want to evaluate programs with strengths in that subspecialty. In addition, it never hurts to have a well-known "name" in a subspecialty write you a strong letter of recommendation. Fellowship directors often trust the strong recommendations of their colleagues, and this can make the difference in competitive fields.

Additionally, it is crucial for all prospective residents—especially those who are thinking about a fellowship—to find out where graduates of a given program are today. This is an appropriate question to ask and is often answered in tabular form during the interview. If not, go ahead and ask; you may not care now, but you'll wish you knew when you apply for some of the more competitive specialties.

Educational Environment

Because residency programs are a form of postgraduate education, you will need to appraise the educational philosophy and facilities at the institutions that interest you. Try to obtain as much information as possible regarding education program Web sites and during interview days. Pay attention to the following aspects of residency programs:

People learn in different ways; make sure you understand your own preferences.

Curricula/conferences. Residents depend on well-organized conferences and teaching rounds to expand their knowledge base and reinforce what they already know. Most programs have developed an organized curriculum that exposes residents to all major topics in the specialty during their training. This curriculum might include rotations, conferences, and syllabi with assigned reading. Within some specialties, there is a lot of variation in emphasis and formality, so you have to decide which combination best fits your needs. For example, some family practice programs emphasize obstetrics while others practically exclude it. Some medicine programs feature heavy experience and training in HIV; others have next to none.

Faculty teaching. The teaching residents receive, as well as the rapport they establish with faculty, can be correlated with many factors, including faculty-to-resident ratio, program setting, the proportion of private attendings, and overall program size. A large program cannot provide as much personal mentoring, but thankfully, you are less at the mercy of a few quirky personalities. When you visit a program, get a sense of how invested the faculty are in the training of its house staff. Also try to get a feel for how important teaching is to the residency program as a whole. Finally, determine if there is an established system for feedback/evaluation of residents and find out how responsive faculty are to this feedback.

Research and teaching opportunities. Research and teaching opportunities are almost essential for those who are planning an academic career or subspecialty training, and such opportunities are desirable even if you do not plan to stay within academic walls. So when you assess the research opportunities at a program, ask yourself the following questions: Are well-established researchers available to guide residents? Is time allotted for research, either as a requirement or as an elective? How successful has the program been in securing grants, hospital funding, or internal funding for research? How satisfied are the residents who are currently completing projects? Or, for that matter, how many dissatisfied residents cite a lack of institutional financial support?

Work Environment

Don't forget to survey the working environment when you size up a residency program. After all, you'll be putting in a lot of hours in that set of buildings with their cast of characters. So don't overlook the considerations outlined below.

Work versus education. Many programs are guilty of exploiting residents' "cheap labor" without providing a rich educational experience. Residency is "learning by doing," to be sure, but be on the lookout for the manner in which service is balanced against education.

Patient population/load. The optimal patient load will provide you with enough clinical experience while still leaving you adequate time and energy to read and attend teaching conferences. Patient load is often a function of the program's setting (see above). On your interview visits, ask for an average patient census and the number of admissions residents get when on call, and discreetly ask residents how they feel about the workload. Also, learn what medical problems are common in the population served by the program. For example, an orthopedics program may get more than its share of trauma cases by virtue of its location near several major highways. You should also try to get a feel for other characteristics of the patient population, such as ethnicity/language (is there a large Spanish-speaking population?), socioeconomic status (urban poor?), and attitude (a typical Saturday night ER crowd?). Keep in mind that the best training environment does not have to match that of your future practice. But you must understand how you learn best.

Patient responsibilities. The whole point of residency training is to provide you with the experience and skills you need to practice medicine unsupervised. So when you visit a program, find out if the attending allows residents to "run the show" or, conversely, if residents need to obtain approval for major decisions. Is backup assistance readily available if the resident or intern needs help?

Call schedule. Call schedules vary widely by specialty, setting, year of training, and training site (for programs with multiple sites). Recognize the range of calls that can deprive you of a good night's sleep. The house officer will often encounter a mix of calls during the year. How much sleep you typically get during a call night and how late you work postcall is almost as important as how often you're on call. For many specialties, call frequency often varies according to training year.

Don't forget to ask about how much protected sleep time you get and when you go home postcall.

Closely tied to call schedule is the number of work hours you will be expected to work per week. With the new resident work-hour legislation in place, residents are not to work more than 80 hours averaged over a four-week period, should have one day off in seven (averaged over four weeks), should have ten hours off between daily duty periods and after in-house call, and should not work more than 30 hours when on call. When on the interview trail, it is important to ask residents how close they come to meeting the 80-hour workweek requirements. In the end, you must determine your threshold and the workload you are willing to tolerate.

Know the new ACGME-mandated resident work-hour guidelines.

Ancillary support. No one is an island, and your team certainly doesn't go it alone in caring for your patients. Good nursing support, consulting services, phlebotomy, laboratory, hospital information services, transport services, and ER care are keys to a smooth clinical work experience. As an intern, you will often be used as a person of last resort to fill any gaps in ancillary support (unless you scut the poor medical student).

Esprit de corps. Esprit de corps is a familiar, albeit foreign, term for morale. To gauge it, trust your intuition as well as your powers of observation. Are the residents "happy campers"? Is the atmosphere friendly or competitive? What kind of camaraderie exists among the residents? Among faculty, house staff, and administration? Look for the answers on your visit by asking the house staff and ancillary staff. Quietly divide and conquer. It is usually easier to get an honest answer in private from a departing resident than to ask the chief resident or the program director in front of 20 other interviewees. Afterward, assess the quality of your own experience during the visit.

Salary

Residents are paid so little that salary is seldom the central issue. Interestingly enough, most of your paycheck comes from the federal government rather than from the program itself, so you may be fattening the bottom line of a hospital that is not even paying you. The average income of an intern in

TABLE 6-5. Average 2005–2006 Resident Stipends

YEAR	ALL	NORTHEAST	SOUTH	MIDWEST	WEST
PGY-1	$41,883	$44,330	$39,707	$41,316	$40,473
PGY-2	43,570	46,265	40,945	42,810	42,934
PGY-3	45,530	48,607	42,522	44,397	45,322
PGY-4	47,271	50,402	43,857	46,163	47,965
PGY-5	49,124	52,094	45,382	48,113	50,567
PGY-6	51,192	54,011	47,223	50,086	53,045

2005–2006 was $41,883, but don't bother calculating your pay per hour; it will only depress you. Salary information is readily available on FREIDA. Your income usually rises incrementally during your residency training, but not by much. It is critical to factor in cost of living when comparing salaries; $30,000 will take you much further in Louisville, Kentucky, than $32,000 in Los Angeles (see Table 6-5).

Moonlighting offers the best of both worlds if you can handle the extra work.

For many, these low figures alone are reason enough to moonlight. Once you are licensed to practice medicine (typically after the first year), you can usually earn anywhere from $20 to $120 per hour working in a variety of settings, including ERs, nursing homes, and outpatient clinics (i.e., "doc in the box" settings); doing insurance company physical exams; and even working in prisons. Some programs actually provide in-house moonlighting opportunities, which can be a crucial source of supplementary income. In-house jobs will often take into account your regular call schedule, making it easier for you to moonlight during residency. On the other hand, many programs either officially ban moonlighting or actively discourage it, so tactfully ask about it on your visit, and someone (usually a graduating resident) will give you the scoop.

Benefits

Key benefits are $ in the bank.

Although everyone remembers to ask about salary, don't forget about other benefits. While benefits should not be the reason you choose to rank a program highly, you should think carefully about a program whose benefits are below the norm. Many programs offer medical insurance, dental services, paid drug prescriptions, employee health services, and psychiatric counseling (see Table 6-6). So shop around carefully, especially if you have a family. You should also be aware that certain benefits at some programs are available only if a resident pays a portion of the cost. You don't want to end up spending part of your meager salary on benefits that other programs would have provided for free. So when you evaluate insurance, ask yourself (1) who is covered (i.e., family); (2) what is covered; and (3) what costs you will have to pay out of pocket.

In addition to asking about health benefits, you should ensure that a program offers adequate life, disability, and liability insurance. After four years in med-

TABLE 6-6. Survey of Health Benefits Offered by Residency Programs

BENEFIT	% FULLY PAID (RESIDENT/ FAMILY)	% OFFERED/COST SHARED (RESIDENT/ FAMILY)	% OFFERED/NOT PAID (RESIDENT/ FAMILY)	% NOT PAID (RESIDENT/ FAMILY)
Group medical insurance	38.5/26.6	61.5/70.6	0/0.5	0/2.3
Group dental insurance	32.1/19.5	51.1/58.8	4.1/4.5	12.7/17.2
Vision	14.9/11.8	32.7/33.3	39.6/31.4	21.8/23.5
Drug prescriptions	29.4/2.9	67.7/26.5	0/2.9	2.9/67.7
Psychiatric benefits	25/15	70/75	25/5	5/5
Counseling	42.9/28.6	50/57.1	7.1/14.3	0/0

ical school and untold thousands of dollars in expenses, you (and your family) don't want to be left high and dry if you get sick or have an accident.

If you're planning to start a family during residency training, scrutinize the rules on maternity/paternity leave (see Table 6-7). Find out if the policy is written or if it varies with each case (and personality). Currently, of course, maternity leave policies tend to be more generous than paternity leave policies. Other benefits to consider include parking, housing, meals, vacation, ed-

TABLE 6-7. Issues Addressed by a Complete Parental Leave Policy

Differences in maternal versus paternal leave policies
Duration of leaves allowed before and after delivery
Which category of leave credited
Whether leave is paid or unpaid
Whether provision is made for continuation of insurance benefits and the payment of premiums
Whether sick leave and vacation time may be accrued from year to year or used in advance
Whether make-up time will be paid
Policies for adoption
Whether schedule accommodations are allowed

TABLE 6-8. Survey of Nonhealth Benefits Offered by Residency Programs

BENEFIT	% FULLY PAID	% OFFERED/ COST SHARED	% NOT OFFERED	% NOT PAID
Life insurance	79.6	11.3	2.3	6.8
Disability insurance	71.8	9.5	9.1	9.5
Housing	0	0	93.1	6.9
Parking	48.3	6.9	13.8	31.0
Meals at work	10.4	31.0	31.0	27.6
On-call meals	58.6	37.9	3.5	0

File PEWs into your manila-folder system after your visit.

ucation leave for conferences, library services (e.g., photocopying), and child care (see Table 6-8).

HOW DO I ORGANIZE THIS INFORMATION?

Great—you know what to look for. But now you need to be able to organize and evaluate all the data. You are already receiving information from multiple sources: from FREIDA, your adviser, and house officers at your medical institution. You will be flooded with even more information on your visits to the programs. All of this information should be going into your centralized manila-folder command center. Additionally, we've included a Program Evaluation Worksheet (PEW) that should allow you to organize information conveniently and evaluate a program objectively (see Figures 6-3A and B and Appendix C). Make a copy for each program on your application hit list, and take these copies with you on the interview trail to record notes and impressions.

After this information has been gathered and organized, remember that programs can change rapidly—in many instances, for the worse. All the preparation in the world cannot prevent you from matching at a program whose director suddenly wins the lottery and moves to Tahiti or whose call rooms are flooded by a natural disaster. But a little luck, a thick skin, and a healthy amount of patience will get you through any situation you encounter.

Factor	Comments
Location	
Setting	
Reputation	
Stability of program	
Subspecialty strengths	
Education	
Conferences/rounds	
Faculty teaching	
Postresidency plans of graduates	
Research/teaching opportunities	
Work Environment	
Patient population/load	
Patient responsibilities	
Call frequency/ hours per week	
Ancillary support (e.g., nursing)	
On-call support (e.g., night float, admission caps)	
Health benefits	
Non-health benefits	
Vacation/sick leave/ parenting leave	

Program Name _____

Date of Visit _____

FIGURE 6-3A. Program Evaluation Worksheet (PEW).

Other Factors/Notes	
Gut feeling	
Advantages	Disadvantages

Preliminary Rank

☐ Top third   ☐ Middle third   ☐ Bottom third   ☐ Do not rank

Interview Log

Name/Address	Notes

FIGURE 6-3B.   Program Evaluation Worksheet (continued).

References

AMA Fellowship and Residency Electronic Interactive Database Web site (www.ama-assn.org/ama/pub/category/2997.htm).

American Urological Association Web site (www.auanet.org).

Association of American Medical Colleges. *COTH Survey of House Staff Stipends, Benefits and Funding, 2005.* Washington, D.C., 2005.

Bickel J. Maternity leave policies for residents: an overview of issues and problems. *Acad Med* 64(9):498–501, 1989.

San Francisco Matching Program Web site (www.sfmatch.org).

Steinbrook R. The debate over residents' work hours. *N Engl J Med* 347(16):1296–1302, 2002.

CHAPTER 7

The Application

There are two categories to which most Match applicants will be applying: Electronic Residency Application Service (ERAS) specialties and early Match specialties (neurosurgery, ophthalmology, plastic surgery, and urology). With regard to the former category, your ERAS token should arrive from your school by early August. If you are participating in the early match, you will need to start this process sooner. For all specialties, a complete program application file will consist of several documents or sets of documents that you must assemble, track, and ultimately send off. You will be pulling together the components of this file all summer long and into early fall (see Table 7-1), and you will then be compiling all relevant information either into the file system that you established during the summer or in your dean's office.

HOW DO I ORGANIZE THE PAPERWORK?

For ERAS specialties as well as for many early Match specialties, you will fill out one common application. For non-ERAS specialties, however, each program will have its own set of application requirements, which will be outlined either in the program's cover letter or within the application itself. Some pro-

TABLE 7-1. Common Elements of an Application File

DOCUMENT	FUNCTION	QUICK ADVICE	MORE INFORMATION
Program application	Foundation of application file	Request by early August. Better to get too many than too few. Most programs participate in ERAS.	See pages 135–139
Dean's letter	Compendium of written evaluations compiled by dean of student affairs	Take an active role in helping dean by editing/supplementing content if possible. Clarify any inaccuracies.	See pages 139–142
Letters of recommendation	Written testimonials from faculty familiar with your work	Solicit letters no later than August. Confirm that writer feels comfortable writing a "strong" letter.	See pages 142–144
Transcript	Academic record	Proofread an unofficial copy before having them sent out.	See page 144
CV	Summary of your credentials, activities, and accomplishments	Pull together by July. Nice to have for preparing personal statement and to accompany requests for letters of recommendation.	See Chapter 8
Personal statement	Opportunity to establish your own voice and distinguish yourself from other applicants	Finish personal statement before applications arrive. Multiple reviewers and revisions are key.	See Chapter 9

THE APPLICATION

grams will ask you to complete the National Resident Matching Program (NRMP) Universal Application, while others will include their own forms. Some programs will want to receive your undergraduate transcript in addition to your medical school transcript. To help you keep track of who wants what, you should photocopy enough copies of the worksheet for application requirements to list all the programs to which you are applying (see Figure 7-1 and Appendix B).

Use a worksheet (like ours) to organize the application process.

Fortunately, there are two steps you can take to prevent paperwork from spiraling out of control: (1) do not add any new programs to your list after you have started working on your applications; and (2) try to complete one item (e.g., obtaining transcripts) for all applications at the same time.

WHO EVALUATES MY APPLICATION?

As you assemble your application materials, be sure to remember your audience. The residency selection committee is usually composed of the resi-

Directions: Fill in blanks below with requested numbers/names/dates. Under **Application Requirements**, list each requirement by name. Once you have assembled the item for that application, check it off.

Program Name	Application Mailing Address	Contact & Phone #	App. Deadline	Application Requirements	Notes
				☐ ☐ ☐ ☐ ☐	
				☐ ☐ ☐ ☐ ☐	
				☐ ☐ ☐ ☐ ☐	
				☐ ☐ ☐ ☐ ☐	
				☐ ☐ ☐ ☐ ☐	

FIGURE 7-1. Worksheet for application requirements.

dency director, several faculty members, and a few house officers. All are **extremely busy people** who would rather be doing something other than screening your application on a Saturday afternoon. So try to make their job as pleasant as possible by submitting a neat, professional-looking application with clear, succinct answers.

Although faculty members are indeed important, you should bear in mind that departmental administrators and administrative assistants can make or break an application. Many students make the mistake of forgetting their manners when scheduling interviews and asking administrative personnel for further information. Not only is this rude, but it could prove to be detrimental to your application, as the comments made by administrative personnel may well influence the committee's impressions of you. Additionally, the departmental administrator often compiles the list of applicants to be interviewed using screening criteria such as board scores and medical school attended. Therefore, it is not difficult for such people to move your application into the "Do Not Interview" pile or, conversely, from that stack into the "To Be Interviewed" pile. If the departmental administrator likes you well enough, he or she may actually push for your application or direct it to a receptive committee member. If you miss any deadlines, friendly administrative assistants may bend rules to keep your application in the running. Administrative personnel also coordinate complexities such as couples applications and visa issues for international medical graduates (IMGs). We could go on, but you get the message!

HOW DO THEY EVALUATE MY APPLICATION?

Once your application lands on the desk of the program director, he or she will direct its contents to a number of readers at different phases in the evaluation process. The typical process can be divided into several stages: screening, the interview, and ranking sessions. Each stage is described below and in subsequent chapters.

Screening

In the initial phase of the evaluation process, your application is usually reviewed by a select few committee members, most of whom screen applications after hours during the week or on weekend afternoons. At this point, some oversubscribed residencies in competitive specialties employ the help of an administrative assistant to divide the applicant pool into a few tiers on the basis of United States Medical Licensing Examination (USMLE) scores or, if available, class rank. Optimally, screeners will read your application, your letters of recommendation, selected portions of your dean's letter, and your transcript. In reality, however, they will likely just scan the highlights of your application package. This is where it can pay off to have an organized CV and a well-written personal statement.

When the committee looks at a dean's letter, members typically focus on junior and senior clerkship evaluations in their field and scan the summary paragraph for crucial code words. Note that the personal statement tends to carry little or no weight at this point in the process, since screeners generally have another 50 files or so to plow through. Screeners then complete an evaluation form, which will toss your application into one of three piles: a recommendation to interview, maybe interview, or not interview. Some programs grant interviews on a rolling basis, so again, it's best to get your application in as early as possible.

The Interview

Many conscientious interviewers will review your file before your actual interview takes place. Others, however, prefer to review your file while you're sitting in their office, which is likely to be distracting when you're already under stress. This behavior is difficult to justify, but get over it. Interviewers will still rank you high or low depending on what they think of this meeting.

Don't let a poorly prepared interviewer throw you off on interview day.

Busy interviewers zoom in on areas that consistently yield the most informational "bang for the buck," such as your CV, transcript, letters of recommendation from well-known writers, and the dean's letter. The importance of your personal statement will depend on the individual interviewer and on your specialty. The interview day is covered in detail in Chapter 11.

Ranking Sessions

After you have completed all your interviews, there remains at least one highly charged, exhausting session in which the full committee attempts to rank the candidates they've seen. In many cases, not all interviewed applicants are ranked. It should also be noted that the real committee battles are not fought over names placed high on the rank-order list (ROL), as the top applicants are easy to rank. Rather, committee members will squabble over the names in the middle ground.

In general, two rules are often observed during this final meeting. The first is that each and every member has a "right of refusal" for any candidate. This means that while a favorite faculty member cannot guarantee you a high rank, an enemy in the ranking committee can kill your ranking candidacy. This practice is more common in the smaller, more competitive specialties. Committee members all respect each other sufficiently to take one another's opinions seriously. The second rule is that committee members who are not familiar with your application will usually defer to those who are. This may seem obvious, but it goes a long way toward explaining some of the seeming randomness of the process. If your last name starts with an "A" and the person who interviewed you is 10 minutes late to the meeting, you may have no advocate present at that meeting when your application is discussed. Conversely, if the faculty member who interviewed you loves your application, you may have a better chance. It's not fair, but that's how the game works.

Academic factors are only part of the selection committee's criteria.

As the meeting wears on, application files may be subjected to less balanced assessments. At this point, the committee is likely to overanalyze your personal statement. Anything unusual in your personal statement or in the rest of your application is much more likely to be judged bizarre than to be weighted in your favor. So the bottom line is this: Be smart and assertive, and don't take unnecessary chances.

Selection Factors

Throughout the evaluation process, the selection committee tests its pool of applicants against certain criteria that are important to its program. You may think that all programs want is an applicant who has been elected to AΩA,

TABLE 7-2. **Factors Most Important to Program Directors**

| 1. Attitude |
| 2. Stability |
| 3. Interpersonal skills |
| 4. Academic performance |
| 5. Maturity |

boasts spectacular board scores, and has "honors" plastered all over his or her transcript. In point of fact, however, academic standing is only part of the story. After all, what good is stellar academic performance if an applicant does not interact smoothly with current faculty, house staff, and administration? Program directors want residents who work hard and perform well on a team. According to program directors, the factors most critical to residency committees tend to be personal (see Table 7-2). This is likely due to the long hours and extended period of time the resident-residency relationship involves. Program directors would prefer to teach someone who doesn't know a lot but is ready to learn rather than cope with a smart but unmotivated resident.

Of course, overall academic performance is important. Among the major academic selection factors, grades in the specialty rotation and electives seem to be the most crucial. Although Figure 7-2 may help you put your performance in perspective, you must keep in mind that selection criteria vary substantially from one field to another. For example, psychiatry residency directors rate AΩA membership as only "somewhat important," whereas general surgery residency directors consider this honor to be a "very important" academic selection factor. See Chapter 4, "Your Specialty and the Match," to learn more about the key criteria in your specialty.

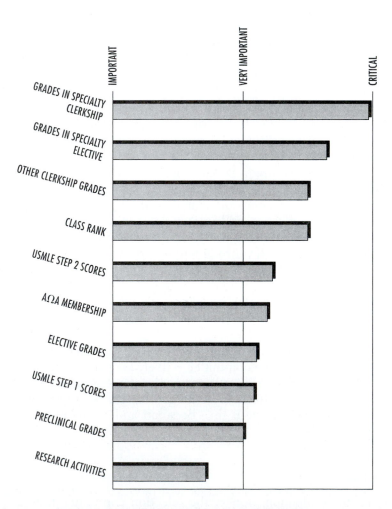

FIGURE 7-2. **Academic factors important to residency directors.**

THE APPLICATION

ERAS Applications

Developed by the Association of American Medical Colleges (AAMC), the Electronic Residency Application Service was first employed in 1995–1996 and has four components that make use of the Internet: the MyERAS applicant Web station, the Dean's Office Workstation, the Program Directors Workstation, and the ERAS Post Office. Using MyERAS, applicants complete their applications, select residency programs, and attach any required supporting documents. ERAS is now entirely online; however, not all aspects of the ERAS application are completed by the student. With ERAS, it is theoretically much easier to keep track of all the documents and forms in your application, as you will always know exactly what went to whom. The intuitive and user-friendly student software automatically guides you through a series of windows to create your application. It's so easy that many students do not even consult the instruction manual (see Table 7-3).

Applicants can use ERAS on any computer (PC or Mac) with World Wide Web access using Netscape 4.77, Internet Explorer 5.0, or AOL 5.0 or greater. In addition, you must have a modem that is 56 kbps or faster, 32 MB of RAM, and an e-mail address. Most medical schools have student computer workstations containing ERAS.

The first step is to create an ERAS account using the "token" supplied to you by your dean's office, usually between late July and August. Once your account has been created, you can start to work on your application. The ERAS application consists of four basic areas: "My Account," "My Application," "My Documents," and "Programs." In "My Account" you will find a profile section, checklist, a section for messages from residency programs, and a password section. The profile is where you enter demographic information, USMLE ID (so scores can be released), ACLS/PALS certification, AΩA membership, and/or Sigma Sigma Phi status. The other sections are all self-explanatory. In "My Application," you essentially enter your CV. Be sure to scrutinize every detail of this document because it is the one document that interviewers will peruse prior to interviews. In addition, once submitted, it cannot be edited. So, you want to be sure it is free of errors! In "My Documents" you create your personal statement and shells for letters of recommendation, and release USMLE/COMLEX transcripts. Further, this section allows you to customize your applications. Moreover, you can individualize your personal statement for each program. Also, you can designate as many letter writers as you would like and assign different letters to different programs. Thus, if one of your letter writers did his residency at a program that you are applying to, you can be sure to send that letter to that program. But keep in mind that you can assign a maximum of only four letters, not including the dean's letter, to any program. Finally, in the "Programs" section you are able to search allopathic/osteopathic programs, select the programs that you would like to apply to, apply to programs (after the September 1 deadline), and visualize and obtain a copy of your invoice. Of note, both your program selection list and the total number of programs to which you are applying are confidential information that remains between you and the dean's office.

Your completed application will then be transmitted to the ERAS Post Office, where your chosen residency programs can download it at any time via the Program Directors Workstation (except for the dean's letter, which is held in

TABLE 7-3. Major Steps in ERAS

Fill out common application form
Create a personal statement
Request letters of recommendation
Release USMLE transcript
Select residency programs to receive applications

THE APPLICATION

the ERAS Post Office until November 1). It is important to note that additional items may be attached to your application as the application process proceeds. For example, if a letter writer has not yet finished writing your letter of recommendation, it can be picked up by the program directors at a later date. The same holds true of programs with late AΩA elections. So **do not let a missing letter of recommendation delay your application!** Simply get the application in and the letters will be added as they come in to the ERAS Post Office.

The ERAS system allows you to create multiple applications for different programs.

ERAS is used by most residency programs in anesthesiology, dermatology, diagnostic radiology, emergency medicine, family practice, general surgery, internal medicine, obstetrics and gynecology, orthopedic surgery, ENT, pathology, pediatrics, physical medicine and rehabilitation, psychiatry, and transitional-year programs. It is also used by all Army and Navy GME-1 positions as well as by combined family practice/psychiatry, internal medicine/emergency medicine, internal medicine/family practice, internal medicine/pediatrics, internal medicine/psychiatry, and internal medicine/physical medicine and rehabilitation programs. Some programs in the above specialties may not be using ERAS, so you may need to contact these programs separately for applications.

As mentioned earlier, U.S. medical students, including osteopathic students, will receive their ERAS token through their student affairs office. IMGs who are interested in using ERAS should contact the Educational Commission for Foreign Medical Graduates (ECFMG), which acts as the dean's office for foreign graduates. The ECFMG will attach deans' letters, transcripts, and letters of recommendation and will transmit USMLE scores on behalf of IMGs. The ECFMG can be reached at the following address:

> ECFMG/ERAS Program
> P.O. Box 11746
> Philadelphia, PA 19101-0746
> www.ecfmg.org

Canadian medical school graduates interested in applying to U.S. residency programs should contact the Canadian Resident Matching Service (CaRMS) at the address below:

> Canadian Resident Matching Service
> 2283 St. Laurent Boulevard, Suite 110
> Ottawa, Ontario, Canada K1G 3H7
> (613) 237-0075
> www.carms.ca

Don't let the fees discourage you from submitting enough applications.

If you decide to apply to additional programs, you can modify portions of your application for these programs before you send your application to each. Although ERAS imposes an absolute deadline of December 1, be sure to check with the individual programs to ascertain their application deadlines. Applicants can also check the status of their documents via the Applicant Document Tracking System (ADTS). This service tells you which documents a given residency program has "picked up" from the ERAS Post Office.

ERAS/Miscellaneous Fees

ERAS fees. Current ERAS fees are as follows: For each specialty, the application plus up to 10 programs selected will cost $60. An additional $8 will be assessed for programs 11–20, $15 for programs 21–30, and $25 for programs 31 and up (see Table 7-4). IMGs will be charged an additional $75 by the ECFMG, since it will serve as their dean's office.

Miscellaneous fees. Applicants are currently charged a $50 fee for an unlimited number of USMLE/NBME (National Board of Medical Examiners) transcripts, which include your Step 1 and Step 2 scores. Once your request reaches the ERAS Post Office, the NBME will begin processing it within one week. Your Step 2 scores will not be automatically sent to residency programs unless you include a transcript request with your application, send an electronic request separately from the application, or mark the box on the application that automatically sends your updated transcript. If you choose to send Step 2 scores separately, you will have to pay $50 again. Osteopathic applicants may request an unlimited number of COMLEX transcripts to be sent via ERAS for $50 as well.

Registering for the Match

Do not forget to register for the Match if you want programs to find your name when they enter their ROL. The AAMC runs both the application process (ERAS) and the matching process (NRMP), and it would seem obvious that people applying for residency might be interested in matching to one. In point of fact, however, the two processes are separate. To register for the Match, you must enter your AAMC ID and pay $65 to the NRMP at www.nrmp.org/res_match/index.html. This fee allows you to rank up to 15 programs. If you wish to rank more than 15 programs, additional fees will apply when you certify your rank list.

Filling out ERAS forms does not register you for the Match.

San Francisco Match

The San Francisco Match application is handled and processed by the Central Application Service (CAS). Bear in mind, however, that while CAS is mandatory for ophthalmology programs and for some programs in neurology, child neurology, and neurosurgery, it is optional for others. CAS materials are generally sent to registered applicants by early July. The CAS process is similar to that of ERAS in that you fill out one common application. After you obtain one copy of each supporting document, you must mail the entire application packet to CAS. Overnight delivery is recommended so that you can track your document's receipt. The application will then be copied and sent to your selected programs. Application fees are currently $60 total for the first 10 pro-

TABLE 7-4. ERAS Fees

NUMBER OF PROGRAMS PER SPECIALTY	AAMC FEES
Up to 10	$60
11–20	$8 each
21–30	$15 each
31 or more	$25 each

grams. An additional $10 each will be charged for programs 11–20, $15 for programs 21–30, $20 for programs 31–40, and $35 for program 41 and up. For more information, go to www.sfmatch.org. In addition, you will be charged a nonrefundable $100 fee for registration and matching.

The Urology Match is very similar to the SF Match and NMRP. Applicants who wish to pursue careers in urology must register with the American Urological Association ($75 fee). Once they have received their ID number, they can register with ERAS or utilize ERAS to contact programs that do not participate in their services, so that they may request applications. Applicants must keep in mind that the deadlines are earlier than common ERAS deadlines; therefore, they must be on top of things early! However, this means that rewards come early as well. The Match is typically finished by late January. For more information, visit www.auanet.org.

Paper (Non-ERAS) Applications

The NRMP Universal Application was created to simplify the application process for non-ERAS programs. The idea was that you would complete this application once and would then send photocopies of it to programs that accept it. Unfortunately, however, a few programs insist on using their own forms. The writing process for non-ERAS programs can thus be very frustrating, since these "custom" applications, while often differing only slightly from the Universal Application in content, use unique layouts—forcing applicants to go back to their typewriters or word processors for yet another round of cut and paste.

Give them what they want where they want it.

If any of your prospective programs request the Universal Application, **fill it out first,** as much of the material that it calls for will resurface in other application forms. Some students find it helpful to hire a secretarial service to handle the paperwork and produce top-quality, customized application materials. If you are on busy clinical rotations or don't have the skills or compulsiveness to track all the details yourself, these services can preserve your sanity.

When you receive a program application, **make at least two photocopies of the blank application.** Neatly write the necessary information by hand on one of the photocopies before typing on the original. That way, if you mortally mess up the original and have no time to request another, the second photocopy will serve as a backup. As you complete the application, keep the following tips in mind:

■ For information to be filled in on the form itself, use a good electric typewriter with good error correction. Alternatively, if you are experienced and ambitious, you may elect to use a word processor. This second method involves the risky process of feeding applications into laser printers or photocopiers (the overlay method)—a true test of your alignment skills. Word processing is best reserved for the personal statement, for which looks count and a nice, proportionally spaced computer font is more compact and readable than most typewriter fonts. If you can't do it right, get help from a computer-savvy friend or a secretarial service.

■ Avoid filling a blank on an application with "See CV" or "See Personal Statement." These abbreviations may make sense to you but can annoy residency directors to no end, since the personal statement or CV is often a loose piece of paper located elsewhere in your application file. In addition, these shorthand terms bespeak a certain lack of motivation. You can, of course, abbreviate specific titles or similar terms in the information requested if necessary (e.g., "U" for "University," "Schl" for "School"). If the space provided is too small, fill it in with the most important information; only then should you add "Also see CV" or "Also see Personal Statement."

- When you are finished, **make and file a photocopy of the complete application.** Applications do get lost in the mail, so you might need to fax a copy or send a replacement by express mail to the program if the post office fouls up. Also, having your copy handy right before your interview serves as a helpful memory refresher. Reviewing what you wrote in your application will help you anticipate questions while also eliminating possible inconsistencies between what you put down on paper and what you may say in person.

If a program that ranks high on your list gives you the choice of the NRMP Universal Application or its own form, use the latter. Resist the urge to take the easy way out, especially if a program expresses a preference for its own application form.

THE DEAN'S LETTER

As we mentioned earlier, the letter from your dean is a key item at the screening and interview stages of the application process. Deans' letters convey a range of information about you to committee members (see Figure 7-3). Although the dean's letter is supposed to be an objective evaluation of your medical school performance, most deans' letters come across as enthusiastic letters of recommendation, thus bolstering many average or weak applications while possibly diluting strong ones. For this reason, the dean's letter is often used less as an objective criterion than as a way to get to know you as an applicant. This is the only document that brings together the diverse experiences that have made up your medical school career.

Although deans' letters can vary substantially, they typically contain the following components:

- **Personal background information.** This includes pertinent and noteworthy information from your undergraduate career and medical school application (e.g., graduating magna cum laude, leadership positions).
- **Preclinical evaluations.** This section will tell the committee about your preclinical honors or, conversely, about any irregularities in progress or required remediation.
- **Clinical evaluations.** This is typically the longest portion of the dean's letter. The majority of deans' letters will include quotes from your clinical evaluations. Some letters cite such evaluations verbatim, while others use abridged versions or just choice positive excerpts. Some deans' letters include histograms that depict the grade distributions in courses and rotations, with the student's position marked on each.
- **Special activities.** Here the dean has an opportunity to highlight your extracurricular activities and any outstanding achievements. These passages often read like portraiture or—at worst—caricature.
- **Summary paragraph.** This section is usually the one that the residency selection committee reads first. It is typically a concise synopsis of the dean's letter and often provides a comparative analysis of your performance, whether through a class rank, a class percentile, or buzzwords that function to cluster or single out students (see Table 7-5).

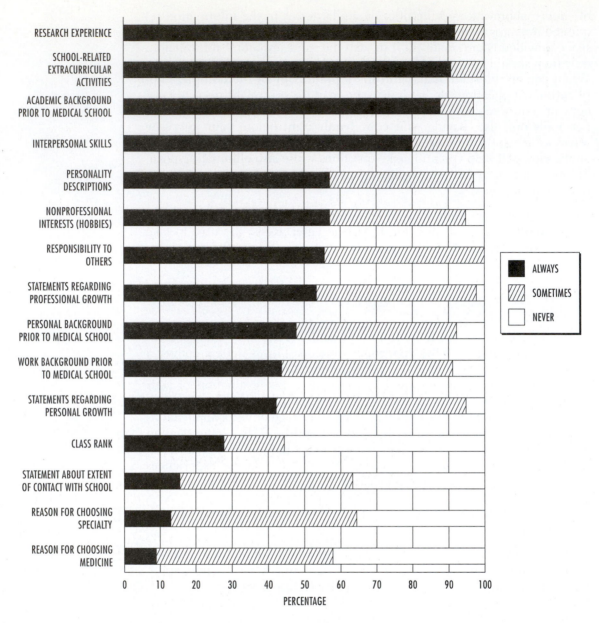

FIGURE 7-3. Information that commonly appears in deans' letters.

Be aware of the level of input

you have into the dean's

letter!

In some cases, the dean's letter can be written without your input. At the other extreme, your school might ask you to proofread the letter for typos and factual errors or even allow you limited editorial privileges with regard to its content. Other schools will consider it a federal offense if you so much as sneak a peek at your dean's letter. If your dean's office calls you in for a talk with the dean, be sure to bring along your CV or personal statement. In any event, ask savvy seniors and your student affairs office about the structure of the typical dean's letter from your institution and try to find out what role you can expect to play in its final development. Table 7-6 presents a tongue-in-cheek view of the code words found in the dean's letter.

If you are given an opportunity to review your dean's letter, check it carefully for accuracy, grammar, and spelling as well as for the presence of all your

TABLE 7-5. Examples of Buzzwords Used in Deans' Letters

Best	Recommend in highest terms	Outstanding	Strongest of year
	Recommend very highly	Excellent	Very strong
	Recommend highly	Very good	Strong
Worst	Recommend	Good	Good

TABLE 7-6. The "Unofficial Guide" to Translating the Dean's Letter[a]

WHAT THE DEAN SAYS	WHAT THE DEAN REALLY MEANS
Sensitive	Cries easily
Very sensitive	Cries on rounds
Very cooperative	Easy; will work extra nights
Relatively good	Wouldn't want him/her for my doctor
Sensitive to patients' needs	Steals food from their trays
Extremely capable	A little better than average
Well-liked	His/her mom always spoke well of him/her
Extremely conscientious	Probably paranoid
Assertive	A real SOB
Self-motivated	Obnoxious
Outstanding integrity	On parole; is watching every step
Enthusiastic	Hebephrenic
Grasps new concepts quickly	Basically stupid, but flexible
Highly satisfactory	Extremely average
Compulsive, goal-oriented	Obnoxious, but no more than average
Recommend with confidence	Glad to get him/her out of our school
Recommend with reservation	Glad to get him/her out of our school
Look forward to watching this individual mature in his/her career	Sure hope the fool improves
Will be an asset to your program	Don't call us, we'll call you!

[a] Adapted from the *New England Journal of Medicine.*

clerkship evaluations (there is no need to point out any weak ones that might be missing). If you have not already done so, do not hesitate to visit your dean of students to discuss any evaluations that you believe to be unfair, inaccurate, or even inappropriate. If your school gives you the opportunity to edit the content of your dean's letter, **grab it!** Medical schools want their graduates to do well, and few can market you as well as you can. Make sure the dean's letter emphasizes your strong points while tactfully expressing concern about negative material that may have made its way into the collection. Everyone has suffered a premature or harsh judgment made by someone who doesn't really know them. If you have one or two isolated "pans" in your record, a sympathetic dean may be willing to soften or delete them. You would much rather have your dean's letter be bland than negative.

Many deans swear that they are not "ranking" students with the last paragraph of the dean's letter. If you have some editorial privileges as to the final version of your dean's letter, this is the place to use them. Tell the dean that if no ranking is being done, you would rather be referred to as "outstanding" than "good" if it's all the same to him or her. At least it's worth a try.

Most deans' letters are mailed out on November 1, a date agreed upon by the Council of Deans. A few deans send out their information earlier. The dean's letter will automatically be attached to your application at this time, not beforehand. You don't have to do much about it other than wait and check the ADTS in early November to verify that it has been picked up by your programs.

LETTERS OF RECOMMENDATION

Along with your dean's letter, your letters of recommendation are vital to the success of your application. You should thus take the time to select your letter writers wisely and provide them with all the materials they may need to refresh their memories when they write their recommendations.

When Should I Start Requesting Letters of Recommendation?

Always meet with your letter writers in person before they write the letter.

You can ask for letters of recommendation after you have completed any significant clinical or research experience. Most students start collecting letters during the third year of medical school. If you did well on a third-year clerkship, ask the attending to write a letter while you are still fresh in his or her mind, keeping in mind that the letter can subsequently be modified to reflect your specialty choice and career goals. In general, whenever you ask for a letter, give the writer at least four weeks to write and mail it off. Treat a letter writer the way you yourself would want to be treated: Supply him or her with your CV, your personal statement, envelopes, and postage. Note that if you are participating in ERAS from a U.S. or Canadian medical school, your dean's office will likely receive and scan these letters into ERAS for you. If you make it easy, the letters are more likely to get done accurately and on time.

How Do I Get a Strong Letter of Recommendation?

When you solicit letters of recommendation, there are a few steps you can take to maximize your chances of getting the strongest possible response.

First, go to the clerkship office and read the evaluations that your potential reference wrote about you during your rotation. The strength and eloquence of the writer's evaluation will certainly be reflected in any subsequent letter he or she may write on your behalf.

Second, when asking for a letter of recommendation, phrase your request carefully. This precaution may reduce your vulnerability to weak letters. Tact and discretion are even more important late in the game, when clerkship evaluations may not be available to you. You can, for example, ask the person, "Do you think you know me well enough to write me a strong letter of recommendation?" If the potential reference does not feel comfortable writing a strong letter about you, he or she can take the graceful exit you provided by saying, "Actually, I don't believe I know you well enough. Perhaps you should ask someone else." Then you are free to request a letter from another attending or faculty member who may give you a better reference.

Third, meet in person with the writer **before** he or she sits down to compose the letter so that you can discuss your choice of specialty and your career goals. Provide your letter writer with a copy of your personal statement, your CV, and the names of the programs you will be considering if it is possible to do so. Medicine is a small world, and many people know one another; your letter writer may be old friends with a few of the program directors you will encounter on your interview trail. If a letter writer cannot meet you despite your reasonable best efforts, you might not get the strongest letter and may consider someone else who can make the time.

Some attendings will draft a letter of recommendation and offer you the chance to read it and either decline or accept it. If the letter is not as strong as you had hoped, you may decline it as long as you have better letters coming (see Table 7-7). If the attending does not offer to show you the letter, you may tactfully try the direct approach and ask if he or she would mind if you saw it.

TABLE 7-7. Signs of a Strong or Weak Letter

STRONG	WEAK
Typewritten on official letterhead and personally signed	Handwritten on plain paper and photocopied
Handwritten postscript a big plus	Signed by an assistant or signature photocopied
Lengthy	Short
Detailed description of fund of knowledge, clinical skills, and past performance	Vague; focuses on marginally relevant personality traits or work habits (e.g.,"He was punctual and well dressed.")
Frequent personal references	Lack of familiarity
Unconditional praise	Lukewarm praise; qualifications of any kind (*but, except,* etc.)

Alternatively, you may opt to be less direct and ask to receive a copy for your files. Many writers view this as a reasonable request, since letters of recommendation often get lost, and you may end up having to fax a copy of the missing letter to the program at the last minute to complete your file. If you are applying in a competitive specialty or if you are a marginal candidate, you may also want to keep copies of your letters for the Scramble in the event that you do not match. Despite all this, some attendings maintain that their letters should remain strictly confidential. If you do see the letter early and it is unfavorable (see Table 7-7), you may decide to withhold program addresses. However, make sure you have someone else to ask for a letter. Even if your letters have been sent, you should be aware of their content just in case an issue pops up during the residency interview.

Whom Should I Ask for Letters of Recommendation?

There are a number of characteristics you should look for in each of your letter writers. If possible, he or she should be someone who:

- Will write you a strong letter
- Knows you well in a clinical setting
- Is well established in the field (in order of desirability: chairman, professor, clinical instructor)
- Works in your specialty choice or in a related field
- Trained at or is well known at your top-choice program

If given the choice between a letter from a well-connected figure who does **not** know you well and one from a lesser-known attending who **is** familiar with you and your work, give priority to the person who knows you better. Unfortunately, many students request letters from less-than-optimal sources (see Table 7-8). Letters from research mentors are acceptable if you already have two clinical letters and have a strong interest in doing research in the future. However, make sure the letter is from someone with whom you have done considerable work (i.e., more than one summer). Letter selection also depends on the type of program to which you are applying. Although it borders on excessive, some applicants actually pick and choose from among five or more letter writers, depending on the characteristics of each program on their list.

TABLE 7-8.
Suboptimal Sources for Letters of Recommendation

Residents
Preclinical professors
Family, friends
Community figures
Previous employers

THE APPLICATION

TRANSCRIPTS

Before you have your medical school and, in some cases, undergraduate transcripts mailed out, request a student copy to review for errors and completeness. You can often obtain an unofficial transcript from your school's Web site. Try to get your official transcript requests to the registrar's office a few weeks before you send out your applications (September for most NRMP applicants). If you receive excellent grades after the transcripts have been mailed, send out updated transcripts.

PHOTO

Most applications as well as ERAS reserve a space for a passport-size photograph. Others will ask you to bring a photo when you interview. Although it is illegal to require a photograph with the application, it is better to comply unless you bear a striking resemblance to Darth Vader. Consider going to a studio for professional photography, and have color prints developed unless specified otherwise. If the pictures turn out well, you can send a 5-by-7 copy to your parents, your significant other, or American Idol!

APPLICATION STATUS

ERAS applicants can track the status of their applications through the ADTS. The ADTS will show you a list of your selected programs along with the dates the documents were uploaded by the dean's office and downloaded by the residency program. Early Match applicants will receive a letter from CAS detailing the documents it has received and the programs to which the application has been sent.

Proofread your transcript; it may contain errors.

Non-ERAS residency programs have a variety of methods for acknowledging receipt of your application material, ranging from no response at all to a letter acknowledging receipt of the application form that checks off any missing materials. Overall, it's up to you to track your application materials. This can easily be done by including a stamped, self-addressed postcard that notes receipt of your application and includes a checklist for missing material (see Figure 7-4). To ensure that the acknowledgment postcard does its job, make arrangements for all other materials well before you send in your applications. The exception is the dean's letter, which is usually mailed out on November 1.

Unfortunately, enclosing a postcard works only if the overworked program secretary is in the mood to mail it back. Return-receipt service from the post office and express mail with tracking numbers are better but more expensive ways to track your applications. If you prefer, wait a few weeks after your application has been sent in, and then call the program to check on your file (especially if you did not receive an "application completed" postcard). Not only will the contact person at the program verify if your file is complete, but he or she may have advance word on your interview status. Most programs don't mind a phone call as long as your manner is courteous and professional. Re-

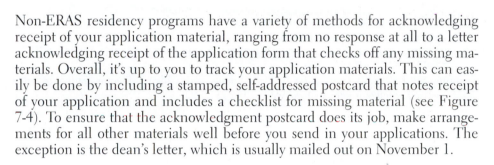

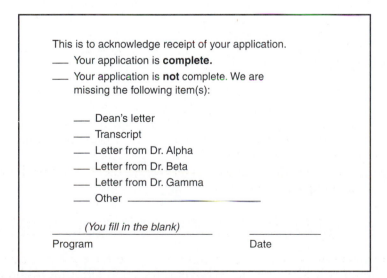

Do not expect programs to notify you of missing materials. Double and triple check yourself.

FIGURE 7-4. **Sample application status postcard.**

member: The impression you make on the office staff may tip the balance toward or against your application.

References

AAMC-ERAS Web site (www.aamc.org/students/eras/start.htm).

Greenburg AG, Doyle J, McClure DK. Letters of recommendation for surgical residencies: what they say and what they mean. *J Surg Res* 56(2):192–198, 1994.

Hunt DD, MacLaren CF, Scott CS, Chu J, Leiden LL. Characteristics of dean's letters in 1981 and 1992. *Acad Med* 68(12):905–911, 1993.

Leiden LI, Miller GD. National survey of writers of dean's letters for residency applications. *J Med Educ* 61(12):943–953, 1986.

San Francisco Matching Program Web site (www.sfmatch.org).

Vanderbilt School of Medicine Guide to Residency Applications. Nashville, TN: Vanderbilt University, 1994.

Wagoner NE, Suriano JR. Program directors' responses to a survey on variables used to select residents in a time of change. *Acad Med* 74(1):51–58, 1999.

Wagoner NE, Suriano JR, Stoner JA. Factors used by program directors to select residents. *J Med Educ* 61(1):10–21, 1986.

Zagumny MJ, Rudolph J. Comparing medical students' and residency directors' ratings of criteria used to select residents. *Acad Med* 67(9):613, 1992.

THE APPLICATION

CHAPTER 8

The Curriculum Vitae

Medicine, like many other fields, values experience. From getting into medical school to gaining chairmanship of your department, much of what you will achieve in medicine will be a direct result of what you have already achieved in the past. These achievements are traditionally chronicled in the curriculum vitae, or CV.

The CV is the bullet presentation of your application.

In the world of applications and interviews, the CV is the equivalent of the one-minute bullet patient presentation: It should be concise yet complete. A well-written CV places a succinct summary of your academic, career, and extracurricular accomplishments at the fingertips of the residency director. The CV is embedded in the Electronic Residency Application Service (ERAS) application, and it works with the rest of your application to win you an interview. After that, the rest is up to you.

During May or June, you should create a preliminary CV so that your letter writers can use it as a reference while they write. You will also want it as you work on your personal statement. You can fine-tune and expand your CV at the end of the summer. This evolving document will then serve as the template for the CV you enter into ERAS in the fall.

As mentioned above, ERAS requires that applicants enter CV information directly into the program without the option to change fonts, styles, or margins. However, there are many reasons why you should create a professionally formatted CV. First, most letter writers will require a CV that they can use as a reference. Second, when you are attending interviews, it never hurts to have a copy in case an interviewer wants to glance at it. So even though you cannot include your personally designed CV as part of your initial application, you should still create an organized, professional, and attractive document. Students applying to specialties whose Match processes lie outside the National Resident Matching Program (NRMP), such as neurology, neurosurgery, ophthalmology, and urology, will use their CV as a part of their application, since they will not be applying through the ERAS program.

WHAT'S IN A CV?

A CV typically will include the following elements:

- **Name and address.** Stick with the same name that you use in your applications, dean's letter, transcripts, and correspondence with programs and the matching service. Make sure you include an address, a phone number, and an e-mail address through which program directors can reach you during the entire interview season. Give a secondary address and phone number (e.g., that of your parents) if no one is at your primary address when you are away during the interviewing season.
- **Objective.** This should consist of a terse, one-sentence statement of your residency and career goals. An objective should be included **only** if your career goals are not readily apparent to the residency director (e.g., a fellowship and academic practice in hand surgery after a residency in orthopedic surgery).
- **Education.** List all major or medically related educational experiences from the present through college. Dual graduate degrees (e.g., MD/PhD, MD/MPH, MD/JD) are particularly impressive and should be highlighted. Include the name and place of the institution, your area of study, dates of enrollment, type of degree received, and honors bestowed at grad-

Start early! Preliminary CVs can help letter writers!

uation (e.g., graduating cum laude). If you are a senior medical student in the United States, list your expected graduation date.

- **Honors.** Include any awards and scholarships that you have received during your med school years as well as the most important awards and scholarships you received during your undergraduate years. If you did well in school or on the boards, list your honors, GPA, class rank, and/or board scores.
- **Publications.** Catalog any abstracts and papers you have published or submitted for publication. Format each publication as a detailed bibliographic reference. Also list research presented or talks given at conferences or poster sessions.
- **Extracurricular activities.** Include the most important long-term activities in which you were involved during medical school (or more recently if you have already graduated). This category should include activities such as community service projects, committee work, and participation in student organizations.
- **Work experience.** List all major or medically related work experiences, whether paid or volunteer (e.g., paramedic work, nursing). Include dates of work experience. Leave the summer job at the country club out.
- **Personal information.** List hobbies and interests that define you. Also mention any special qualifications or skills that might enhance your effectiveness as a house officer (e.g., foreign language training, knowledge of American sign language, computer skills).
- **Professional memberships.** Be sure to mention professional organizations to which you belong (e.g., American Academy of Pediatrics).

The phrase "references available upon request," seen in most nonmedical CVs, is redundant in medicine, since letters of recommendation are a required element of the application. Sometimes, however, it helps to list your references by name in the CV, especially if those references are particularly illustrious and widely respected.

Note that certain information is not appropriate for a medical professional CV (see Table 8-1). However, you may have to consider including information about citizenship or visa status if you are an international medical graduate (IMG).

TABLE 8-1.
Information Not Appropriate in a CV
Birthplace and date
Citizenship status (except IMGs)
Marital status
Names of spouse and family members
High school education/ accomplishments

HOW DO I PUT TOGETHER MY CV?

Study the sample CVs starting on page 150 to get a feel for the appearance you want in your finished CV (see Figures 8-1 through 8-4). On a word processor, fill in information under the categories listed above. If you have nothing to say under a category, do not include it. Note that most CVs start with "Name/Address" and "Education" and end with "Personal." In the middle, however, you can rearrange the order of the remaining categories to emphasize strengths and downplay less impressive areas. Refer to the sample CVs to see the various designs that are available.

After you have input this basic information, edit your document into a professional and attractive format and style using the sample CVs as a guide. See Table 8-2 for specific writing tips. You should also make sure your CV is pleasing to the eye (see Table 8-3). Remember to keep your language terse. Use vivid nouns and active verbs to demonstrate strength, enthusiasm, and initiative (see Tables 8-4 and 8-5). Also pay careful attention to style and punctuation. Medicine is a detail-oriented specialty, and sloppiness can be interpreted

Prioritize! Organize your CV to highlight your strengths.

This applicant has a well-rounded CV with no real outstanding achievements. But because he is applying to several academic training programs, he chooses to list his research experience first.

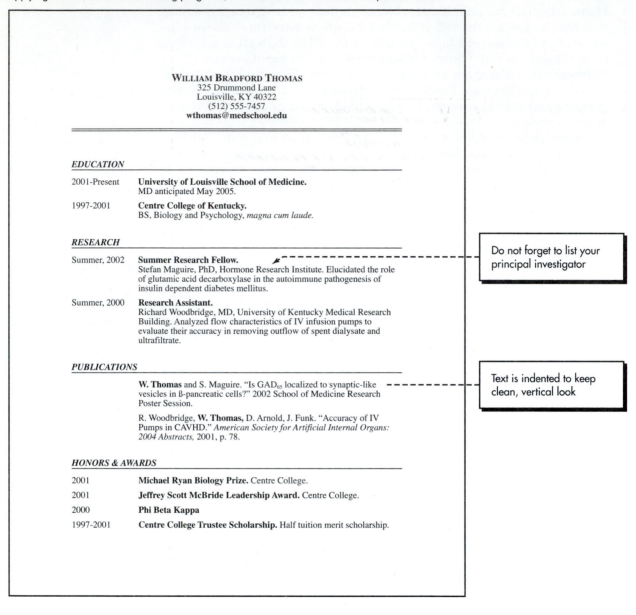

WILLIAM BRADFORD THOMAS
325 Drummond Lane
Louisville, KY 40322
(512) 555-7457
wthomas@medschool.edu

EDUCATION

2001-Present	**University of Louisville School of Medicine.** MD anticipated May 2005.
1997-2001	**Centre College of Kentucky.** BS, Biology and Psychology, *magna cum laude.*

RESEARCH

Summer, 2002	**Summer Research Fellow.** Stefan Maguire, PhD, Hormone Research Institute. Elucidated the role of glutamic acid decarboxylase in the autoimmune pathogenesis of insulin dependent diabetes mellitus.
Summer, 2000	**Research Assistant.** Richard Woodbridge, MD, University of Kentucky Medical Research Building. Analyzed flow characteristics of IV infusion pumps to evaluate their accuracy in removing outflow of spent dialysate and ultrafiltrate.

Do not forget to list your principal investigator

PUBLICATIONS

W. Thomas and S. Maguire. "Is GAD_{65} localized to synaptic-like vesicles in ß-pancreatic cells?" 2002 School of Medicine Research Poster Session.

R. Woodbridge, **W. Thomas,** D. Arnold, J. Funk. "Accuracy of IV Pumps in CAVHD." *American Society for Artificial Internal Organs: 2004 Abstracts,* 2001, p. 78.

Text is indented to keep clean, vertical look

HONORS & AWARDS

2001	**Michael Ryan Biology Prize.** Centre College.
2001	**Jeffrey Scott McBride Leadership Award.** Centre College.
2000	**Phi Beta Kappa**
1997-2001	**Centre College Trustee Scholarship.** Half tuition merit scholarship.

FIGURE 8-1. Sample CV no. 1.

WILLIAM BRADFORD THOMAS

EXTRACURRICULAR

2004-Present   **Faculty Student Network Committee.** Organized events and meetings for faculty advisers and medical students.

               School of Medicine Representative, Registration Fee Committee. Allocated student fees to student organizations and services.

2002-2003   **Peer Counselor, Campus Health.** Provided counseling and support for first-year medical students.

2000-Present   **Homeless Health Clinic.** Evaluated and treated homeless patients as medical volunteer in homeless shelter.

2001-2002   **Vice-president, AMA–Medical Student Section Chapter.** Organized health fairs and guest speakers for medical school chapter.

> Use "action" verbs to give an active tone

PROFESSIONAL MEMBERSHIPS

2001-Present   **American Medical Association, Medical Student Section**

2004-Present   **American Academy of Pediatrics, Medical Student Section**

PERSONAL

               Proficient in American sign language.
Hobbies include volleyball, jogging.

FIGURE 8-1. Sample CV no. 1 (continued).

This CV emphasizes the applicant's considerable research accomplishments. If she were applying to clinical programs, she might choose to highlight her strong extracurricular activities.

Sarah Lin

Permanent Address	*School Address*
P.O. Box 271 MDSC	234 Wisteria Lane
Clarksville, IN 47160	Nashville, TN 37215
(812) 555-3952	(615) 555-5456
	slin@medschool.edu

EDUCATION

Vanderbilt University School of Medicine   *2002 to Present*
Nashville, TN
   MD EXPECTED IN MAY 2006

St. Louis University   *1998 to 2002*
St. Louis, MO
   BA, BIOLOGY AND PSYCHOLOGY, MAGNA CUM LAUDE

RESEARCH

Research Assistant   *Summer 2003*
University of California, San Diego
   SAMUEL STOCKTON, MD, PHD. Developed a rat model to study the
   inflammatory process in asthma.

Research Assistant   *January 2003 to May 2003*
Vanderbilt University School of Medicine
   SHELLEY PISA, MD. Characterized the interactions between anesthetic drugs
   and the erythrocyte B and 3 anion exchange channel.

Research Assistant   *January 2001 to May 2002*
St. Louis University
   ANTHONY HILL, PHD. Explored the medicinal value of the plant *Rhamnacea*
   used by South American Indians in wound healing.

Research Assistant   *September 2001 to December 2002*
St. Louis University
   TIMOTHY ROBERTS, PHD. Developed protocols for the use of mutant
   strains of *Chlamydomonas* in transformation experiments.

> Alternative way to keep dates separated from text

FIGURE 8-2. Sample CV no. 2.

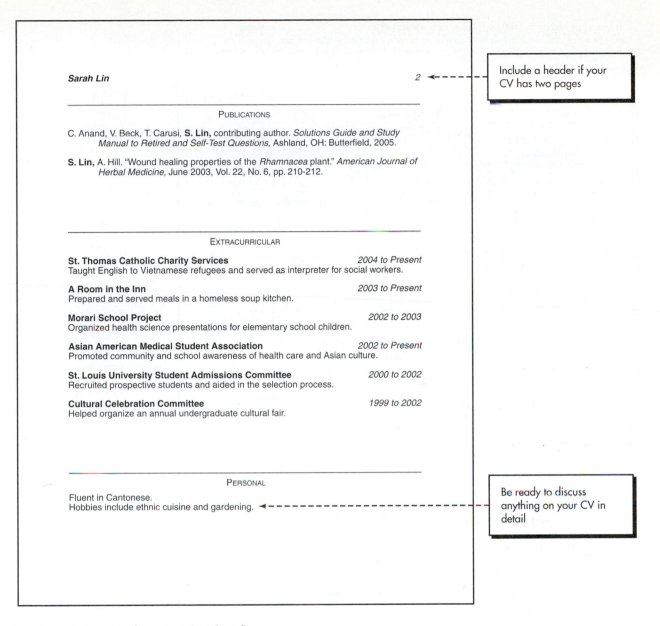

PUBLICATIONS

C. Anand, V. Beck, T. Carusi, **S. Lin,** contributing author. *Solutions Guide and Study Manual to Retired and Self-Test Questions,* Ashland, OH: Butterfield, 2005.

S. Lin, A. Hill. "Wound healing properties of the *Rhamnacea* plant." *American Journal of Herbal Medicine,* June 2003, Vol. 22, No. 6, pp. 210-212.

EXTRACURRICULAR

St. Thomas Catholic Charity Services *2004 to Present*
Taught English to Vietnamese refugees and served as interpreter for social workers.

A Room in the Inn *2003 to Present*
Prepared and served meals in a homeless soup kitchen.

Morari School Project *2002 to 2003*
Organized health science presentations for elementary school children.

Asian American Medical Student Association *2002 to Present*
Promoted community and school awareness of health care and Asian culture.

St. Louis University Student Admissions Committee *2000 to 2002*
Recruited prospective students and aided in the selection process.

Cultural Celebration Committee *1999 to 2002*
Helped organize an annual undergraduate cultural fair.

PERSONAL

Fluent in Cantonese.
Hobbies include ethnic cuisine and gardening.

Include a header if your CV has two pages

Be ready to discuss anything on your CV in detail

FIGURE 8-2. Sample CV no. 2 (continued).

THE CURRICULUM VITAE

This applicant has an impressive number of awards and honors. Because she is entering family practice, she emphasizes her community service experience and lists her research on the second page.

Jacquelyn H. Lemmon

School Address
576 London Road, Apt. #5
Tucson, AZ 85719
(602) 555-7456
jlemmon@medschool.edu

Permanent Address
2145 Red Valley Drive
Danville, TN 37205
(615) 555-5760

Education

2002–2006	UNIVERSITY OF ARIZONA SCHOOL OF MEDICINE
	M.D. expected in May, 2006
1998–2002	WASHINGTON UNIVERSITY
	B.S. in Engineering & Policy

Honors & Awards

2004	BRISTOL-MYERS SQUIBB SCHOLAR
2003–2006	MICROBES AND DEFENSE SOCIETY
2003	DIABETES SUMMER RESEARCH GRANT
	Awarded by Diabetes Research and Training Center.
2003	SUMMER RESEARCH GRANT
	Awarded by American Society for Lasers in Medicine and Surgery.
2002–2006	JUSTIN POTTER SCHOLARSHIP
	Merit award based on leadership potential.
2001–2002	MORTAR BOARD HONOR SOCIETY
1998–2002	JOHN B. ERVIN SCHOLARSHIP

All caps is an alternative to boldfaced text.

Extracurricular

2002–Present	STUDENT NATIONAL MEDICAL ASSOCIATION
	Promoted health care and minority issues. Served as co-chairperson and treasurer of Arizona chapter.
2004–Present	TUCSON CARES
	Made lecture presentations on HIV/AIDS to the general public on behalf of agency, which serves HIV/AIDS population.

FIGURE 8-3. Sample CV no. 3.

Extracurricular, *continued*

2002–Present   SERVICE ACTIVITIES
Participated in several community service activities including Inn for ◄- - - - - - A good way to present
the Homeless, Habitat for Humanity, wheelchair ramp construction,   multiple small activities.
and role model activities for black youth.

2002   SUBSTANCE ABUSE AND PREVENTION PROGRAM
Counseled high-risk youth.

Research

March–August 2005   RESEARCH ELECTIVE, CENTERS FOR DISEASE CONTROL
AND PREVENTION
Preceptor Richard Woodbridge, MD. Designed methods for
collecting and organizing for international importations data.
Collected and analyzed 2005 data with comparison to data collected
from 1996 to 2004.

2004   RESEARCH ASSISTANT
Preceptor George Sherman, MD. Characterized lymphocytic
migration in RSV-infected mice. Results presented at National
Medical Fellowships Research Seminar in February, 2005.

Summer 2003   SUMMER RESEARCH FELLOW
Preceptor Lou Ritter, MD. Tested various pulse structures of the
electron laser to evaluate its efficacy in bone ablation.

Summer 2003   RESEARCH ASSISTANT
Preceptor Lou Ritter, MD. Developed optimal laser firing patterns to
achieve minimal thermal buildup in a collagen-based target. Results
presented to the Arizona Diabetes Research Training Center.

Personal

Hobbies include jogging, playing piano, and swimming.

2

FIGURE 8-3. Sample CV no. 3 (continued).

Both a one-page CV and a two-page CV are acceptable. Because everything is on one page, the order of categories is not as important.

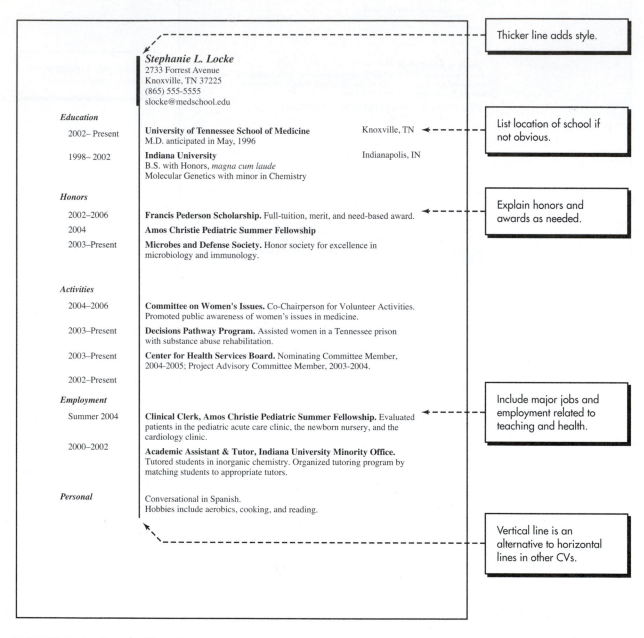

Stephanie L. Locke
2733 Forrest Avenue
Knoxville, TN 37225
(865) 555-5555
slocke@medschool.edu

Education

2002– Present   **University of Tennessee School of Medicine**   Knoxville, TN
M.D. anticipated in May, 1996

1998– 2002   **Indiana University**   Indianapolis, IN
B.S. with Honors, *magna cum laude*
Molecular Genetics with minor in Chemistry

Honors

2002–2006   **Francis Pederson Scholarship.** Full-tuition, merit, and need-based award.

2004   **Amos Christie Pediatric Summer Fellowship**

2003–Present   **Microbes and Defense Society.** Honor society for excellence in
microbiology and immunology.

Activities

2004–2006   **Committee on Women's Issues.** Co-Chairperson for Volunteer Activities.
Promoted public awareness of women's issues in medicine.

2003–Present   **Decisions Pathway Program.** Assisted women in a Tennessee prison
with substance abuse rehabilitation.

2003–Present   **Center for Health Services Board.** Nominating Committee Member,
2004-2005; Project Advisory Committee Member, 2003-2004.

2002–Present

Employment

Summer 2004   **Clinical Clerk, Amos Christie Pediatric Summer Fellowship.** Evaluated
patients in the pediatric acute care clinic, the newborn nursery, and the
cardiology clinic.

2000–2002   **Academic Assistant & Tutor, Indiana University Minority Office.**
Tutored students in inorganic chemistry. Organized tutoring program by
matching students to appropriate tutors.

Personal   Conversational in Spanish.
Hobbies include aerobics, cooking, and reading.

Thicker line adds style.

List location of school if not obvious.

Explain honors and awards as needed.

Include major jobs and employment related to teaching and health.

Vertical line is an alternative to horizontal lines in other CVs.

FIGURE 8-4. Sample CV no. 4.

TABLE 8-2. CV Writing Tips

Organize categories to highlight strengths.
If you're an older applicant, try to avoid unexplained gaps in time line.
Use terse, precise, and vivid language.
Create parallel structure in lists (e.g., each item in a list starts with a verb).
Follow consistent punctuation rules.
Follow consistent capitalization rules.
When in doubt, consult a style manual or a professional editor.

as evidence of carelessness or lack of motivation. If you have any further doubts, refer to the sample CVs, show your draft to a friend with good writing skills, or consult a manual of style such as Strunk and White's *Elements of Style*.

After you have drafted your CV, ask your career adviser and at least one other person to read it and provide feedback on appearance/legibility, ease of reading, grammar, punctuation, and style (see Table 8-3). After making any necessary revisions, print the CV from a laser printer onto high-quality paper.

TABLE 8-3. CV Layout and Design Tips

Allow for generous margins (1–1.5 inches).
Limit CV to two pages.
Avoid splitting a section when going from page 1 to page 2.
Try a serif font (e.g., Times Roman) as the base text font for better legibility. Save sans serif (e.g., Arial) for section headers.
Do not go below 12 points for font size and 14 points for leading.
Stay true to your fonts. Too many can be distracting and gaudy.
Be consistent with section headers in style and formatting.
Boldface your name in any publications cited.
Use boldface, small caps, italics, and bullet symbols sparingly. Avoid underlining.
Print CV on a laser printer at 300 dpi or more.
Print CV on a heavyweight, cotton bond paper. Use a neutral color (e.g., ivory).
Make sure the printed CV photocopies well.

TABLE 8-4. **Action Verbs**

accelerated	directed	lectured	reorganized
accomplished	effected	led	revamped
achieved	elucidated	maintained	reviewed
adapted	established	managed	revised
administered	evaluated	mastered	scheduled
analyzed	examined	motivated	set up
approved	expanded	operated	solved
attained	expedited	organized	streamlined
clarified	facilitated	originated	structured
completed	found	participated	studied
conceived	generated	performed	supervised
conducted	improved	pinpointed	supported
controlled	increased	planned	synthesized
coordinated	influenced	proposed	taught
created	implemented	proved	trained
delegated	initiated	provided	translated
demonstrated	instructed	recommended	used
designed	interpreted	reduced	won
developed	launched	reinforced	wrote

TABLE 8-6.
Appropriate Colors and Patterns for CV Paper

White
Ivory
Beige
Light gray
Flannel pattern
Speckle pattern

Choose a heavy cotton bond paper in white or a neutral color to make your CV stand out in a pile (see Table 8-6). Alternatively, you take the electronic file to a copy center, choose paper that is the appropriate color and bond weight, and print high-quality laser copies on the spot.

If you don't have access to a computer or a printer, don't know how to use one, or just freeze when it comes to putting your life history on paper, you can have your CV created and reproduced by a copy center (e.g., Kinko's) or by a résumé specialist listed in the Yellow Pages or on the World Wide Web.

KISSES OF DEATH

Finally, we are providing you with a handy checklist of "no-no's" for CVs. Any one of these can be a killer. To repeat advice given earlier, have your adviser and another competent person read your CV, paying particular attention to the following:

- **Unprofessional appearance.** Do not write your CV by hand or use a typewriter. Dot matrix is also dead. Laser or inkjet printing at 300 dpi is now the standard; 600 dpi laser output, also readily available, is slightly better.

TABLE 8-5. **Concrete Nouns and Positive Modifiers**

ability	competent	proficient	technical
actively	consistent	qualified	unique
capacity	effectively	resourceful	versatile
competence	pertinent	substantially	vigorous

If you find a mistake on your CV, no matter how minor it may be, print out a new, corrected version. Do **not** make corrections, handwritten or typed, on the CV itself. Use only high-quality, heavyweight bond paper in white or ivory. This is not the time to go "legally blonde" with pastel pink, scented résumé paper. Stick to the basics.

Avoid the colors of the rainbow.

- **Inaccuracies or exaggerations.** Present your talents and accomplishments in the best possible light, but do not misrepresent them. Residency directors have many ways to verify your claims. Even a minor "misrepresentation" can have a major impact on your credibility.

- **Too lengthy.** Do not exceed two pages in length unless you have really stellar experience and an impressive list of publications to justify more space. Remember that this is a capsule summary of your career to date, not an extended autobiography.

- **Misspellings, poor grammar.** These unspectacular mistakes will only contribute to an image of carelessness or incompetence, particularly since word processors make it easy to check spelling and grammar.

- **Weak writing.** Verbosity kills; keep your sentences short and succinct. Specifics count; the more precisely you can describe your experience, the better the reader can picture—and appreciate—what you say. Stay away from bland nouns and passive verbs.

References

"Resume Guidelines." West Springfield, MA: Southworth Paper Company, 1995.

Ireland S. *The Complete Idiot's Guide to the Perfect Resume,* 2nd ed. New York: Alpha Books, 2000.

The Personal Statement

The personal statement is enigmatic; there is little to nothing in the literature that provides information about what program directors think about this part of the application process, how it might help or hurt applicants, or how it is used. That said, several generalizations can be made from comparing experiences with many program directors.

HOW A PERSONAL STATEMENT CAN HELP THE APPLICANT

The personal statement will put a face with the numbers.

As with the personal interview, the personal statement can help applicants declare their total commitment to the specialty for which they are applying. Program directors like to read about an applicant's love for the academic and personal aspects of the specialty. "Here is a student," they will note, "who will never change specialties, who will never become bored by the work, who will always be upbeat and keep colleagues seeing the upside of the field." Students correctly sense that this is a great opportunity to express their goals. Lofty goals and high expectations should thus be encouraged. Program directors know that some idealism will dissipate, that the missionary instinct will meet up with the realities of family life, and that the problems of health care delivery will ultimately prove sobering. However, they have also likely seen how one young physician can indeed change the world and certainly affect a program for the better. So in addition to one's enthusiasm for the profession of medicine and the specialty itself, one's goals, hopes, and predictions for success are generally welcome words to a program director.

WHAT BELONGS IN A PERSONAL STATEMENT?

Medical students can enjoy great moments of clarity, inspiration, and growth while on the wards or clinics. If you have had such an experience, by all means describe it. Keep in mind, however, that exaggerated emotional descriptions will be obvious to the reader; the hug of a grateful child is not a believable reason for choosing pediatrics any more than the first amazing observation of childbirth is a reason for choosing obstetrics. On the other hand, the death of a mother from breast cancer has indeed instilled a lifetime of passion in numerous students who chose to become oncologists. If you are a student who has been influenced by some deep-seated experience, describe it. If not, there is no need to try to create such an experience.

One aspect of the personal statement is for certain: It will be used, like the CV, as a menu for your interview. So do not write about something that you do not want to discuss. If you write that caring for your brother with diabetes has given you deep insight into the disease, be prepared to describe those insights. If a summer research experience showed you the beauty of science, express that beauty in words, but be sure you remember what you actually did in the laboratory!

The personal statement is a time to elaborate on strengths. If you were elected to AΩA, that will be apparent on other aspects of your application. However, if you became an AΩA member and then joined a tutoring group or manned an indigent clinic in the AΩA spirit of serving the suffering, here is an opportunity to bring your achievements to life. Weaknesses do not make good content. Drawing attention to a failed USMLE attempt or to a low clerkship score with an explanation of illness or personal distraction is rarely helpful. Describing oneself as great on the wards but as a poor test taker is also worrisome. The personal statement may be a time to celebrate a great medical school and appreciation for an excellent education. Any experiences that reflect poorly on your school or your education should not be included (e.g., "My shelf exam scores are low because we received no guidance on what to study").

Some students create personal statements that suggest eccentricity. In such cases, the personal statement has the potential to become a self-inflicted wound. It may indeed be exemplary that you climbed Mount Everest, but don't give the impression that you might choose to do so again in the middle of your ICU rotation. Perhaps you won a great political victory in college—but don't make yourself sound like the resident most likely to establish the first residents' union in your hospital.

Some program directors will read your statement quickly and are not likely to evaluate punctuation. However, a poorly written statement replete with spelling mistakes and other errors reflects poorly on the applicant. We are members of a profession that does not tolerate mistakes well. So read and reread your statement, and have others look at it. If your adviser says that it is perfect as is, thank him/her and give it to someone else to review. Then, when you are through with the statement, let it sit for a few days and read it out loud. It will likely require some additional fine-tuning. Length will vary with theme and style, but you should probably not exceed one and one-half pages. See Table 9-1 for additional tips.

The personal statement is unlikely to affect your chances for acceptance in a particular residency, but it is an important statement about yourself at a time of great significance to your career.

Your weaknesses will be apparent from your application. Don't use the personal statement to highlight them.

SAMPLE EXCERPTS

We have included excerpts from actual personal statements as examples of "do's and don'ts" for certain issues. Names and locations have been changed to protect the writers' identities, but otherwise you're reading what the residency directors read. Most of the applicants behind these statements matched at excellent institutions across the country. The comments that accompany our examples are derived from the observations of several residency directors, admissions committee members, and a professional editor. We hope that these critiques will help you acquire a "feel" for good form as well as good content. Keep in mind, however, that no two residency directors (even in the same specialty) read a personal statement with the same opinions and preferences.

Strong or Engaging Openings

Example #1. This applicant in emergency medicine draws on rich family and cultural traditions and values. A residency director reading this introduction is not only making the acquaintance of an applicant, they are learning about the applicant's entire value system.

> My great-grandfather once told me that everyone's life is like a book, full of chapters that are continually written and revised. Each life, each book, is unique, made so through the experiences and the actions of the person living. My personal anthology is no exception, having been enriched by the many people whom I have met. Through these experiences, I have strengthened my desire to enter a training program that will lead to a career in emergency medicine. Thus begins a new chapter in my book.

Careful word choice enlivens an overused analogy.

Excellent transition to background info.

TABLE 9-1. Personal Statement Tips

DO

Get an early start. A well-written statement requires a significant investment of your time and energy.
Have a high-quality draft ready at the time you contact potential letter writers. Most will want a copy of your personal statement.
Catch the readers' attention with a strong opening.
Consider including your motivation for choosing the specialty, your ideal residency program, and/or future aspirations in the specialty.
Highlight your strengths and accomplishments; expand on significant extracurricular and community accomplishments.
Make every word count. Use terse, precise, and vivid language to tell your story.
Keep your audience in mind! Convey the qualities of a good resident to program directors and faculty who will be reviewing your statement.
Remember to make it "flow." Smooth transitions keep your reader engaged.
Make it personal. Consider discussing your interests outside of medicine if they pertain to qualities that will make you a good resident.
Tie it all together with a strong finish.
Limit the length of your essay to about one page. Too short conveys a lack of effort and interest.
Have your adviser, other faculty, and your program director review your statement.
Be familiar with your essay. Any material contained within it is a fair topic for discussion in interviews.

DON'T

Blow it off. You have no way of knowing which programs will weight your statement heavily and which will merely glance at it. Prepare your statement as if every program will read it carefully. An inferiorly written statement can only hurt your application.
Simply recap all of the information in your CV. Pick a few items of significance and expand on them to develop an idea or point central to your strengths as an applicant in your desired specialty.
Use worn-out clichés, metaphors, and analogies.
Start every sentence with "I."
Be shy. Go ahead and express lofty career goals or high expectations (within reason). Programs will admire your future aspirations.
Make excuses. The personal statement is not the place to call attention to weaknesses in your application. Save the explanation of failed boards or a poor clerkship grade for the interview.
Be afraid to be different. Just steer clear of eccentric.
Make grammar and spelling mistakes. These errors demonstrate carelessness, a quality unbecoming of a future resident.
Embellish, inflate, or lie under any circumstances. It is definitely not worth the price you will pay if you are discovered.
Be too verbose. Keep it short, sweet, and to the point. Your audience will thank you.
Come across as arrogant. This is the place to showcase your strengths, but in a humble way.

Example #2. A well-done teaser for the rest of the statement. This family practice applicant weaves his sense of social responsibility and worldview (major family practice values) through a number of vivid experiences. Like a seductive movie trailer, the introduction pulls the reader in for more. The reader is left thinking, "This might be someone who would be fun to work with." The only way they will know for sure is by offering an interview!

> I have always been interested in people's stories. This, and a deep-seated desire to help make the world a better place, have drawn me to the work I do. From working on a crew harvesting filberts to sitting down for a bowl of soup with a homeless friend, I have met many people, each one with a story, each story having something to teach me. Some of the wisest people I have met are very poor with little access to housing, education, or health care. I get a lot out of listening to their stories; what do I give back? I first began to question the ethics of being a responsible listener when I went to Nicaragua as a Spanish interpreter. I was with a group of agronomists on a struggling agricultural cooperative nestled deep in the mountains of Matagalpa. The life was hard, but the work was fascinating and the setting beautiful. I finally got up the courage to ask the cooperative leader if I could stay longer. He smiled, "You gringos eat a lot. Now, maybe if you were a doctor . . ." I chose to become a physician as a way to work intimately with people and hear their stories. But, just as importantly, it is a way to tangibly improve their lives.

| An enticing invitation to any director who has seen too many formulaic statements. |

| Major cliché. |

| A noble reason to become a doctor. But why medicine versus other altruistic vocations? |

Example #3. This applicant in anesthesiology successfully recycles a familiar travel theme with vivid imagery. The opening paragraph introduces a traveler enriched by his adventures. Unfortunately, we begin to sense that his actions have an unsettled, random quality.

> While driving in the Mojave Desert, I turned off Highway 14 onto a dirt path. The road was crisscrossed by many other trails. Small hills blocked my view of what lay ahead on each road. Unable to see what each road led to, I randomly chose to drive along one road, then another, and then another. Every new direction possessed its own beauty and worth. One road revealed towering, sand-carved cliffs with striated bands of crimson, orange, and tan spotted with turquoise. Another road led to a lone Joshua tree standing majestically in the desert grass. Each new path inspired a new thought. I have had a similar experience in medicine.

| One hopes his choice of specialty was more deliberate. Rewrite to show some method to this madness. |

| Vivid! You feel as if you're there. |

| Weak tie-in to medicine. |

Example #4. This applicant in orthopedic surgery wants to return to the Midwest after having trained at an East Coast medical school. He combines the family legacy of an immigrant background with the rustic, traditional values of Middle America. By playing up the Midwest, however, he runs the risk of turning off East and West Coast directors in a highly competitive specialty in which applicants must often apply coast to coast in order to match.

> Growing up in the small farming community of Vernon in east-central Indiana, I have experienced a spectrum of attitudes unique to a rural population. Folks here are down to earth, with simple, relaxed lifestyles. It was here where I have lived almost all my life, moving from Birmingham, Alabama, my birthplace, at nine months of age. It was here where my father set up his urology practice 30 years ago, having come from abroad with little more than a dream for a successful future. It was here, amidst the cornfields and cattle which I could see from my bedroom window, that I grew up with my older sister and younger brother under a strict, coherent value system of hard work, motivation, dedication, and perseverance.

| Back off a little on the rural imagery here. We get the point. |

| Nice way of associating yourself with a set of values. Stating the same directly can come off as presumptuous. |

Reasons for Entering Specialty

Example #1. The following comes close to being a model illustration of good organization and presentation of motivations for pursuing a specialty. The applicant is obviously comfortable discussing the specialty and appears sincere in his enthusiasm without being patronizing. The writing is spare but is neither dry nor flat.

A bit of a cliché.

Note the number of concrete reasons orthopedics appeals to him.

A good paragraph that plays to the classic strengths of the specialty.

I grew up with surgery in my blood, but it was not until the middle of my third year of medical school that I discovered that I wanted to practice orthopedic surgery. It was at this time that I was first exposed to orthopedic surgery at Springfield Memorial Hospital. My love of being in the operating room, combined with the very precise mechanical and technical nature of orthopedic surgery, sparked my interest in the field. Perhaps the feature that fascinates me the most about orthopedics is that it is both a craft and a science. I enjoy the "hands-on" nature of orthopedic surgery, both in clinic and in the operating room. I am also attracted to the diversity of orthopedic cases and the vast amount of direct patient contact. Treating patients of all age groups and both sexes, with a wide variety of problems encountered at work, in accidents, or during recreation, makes orthopedic surgery a very exciting specialty. Above all, although very demanding, I found my orthopedic surgery experiences to be the most rewarding and exhilarating in medical school. One can almost always do something specific and helpful for each patient, usually leading to a complete resolution of the patient's problem, so they can resume an active lifestyle.

Example #2. This is a tightly written paragraph in which the applicant clearly delineates her reasons for entering the specialty. The writing is fast-paced and precise, like the specialty she aspires to enter.

Poor word choice. ER docs should be cool under fire.

Text flows well.

Although I have found all my clinical rotations interesting, I experienced the most excitement from my time in the emergency department. Emergency medicine offers me the opportunity to be at the forefront of medicine and to participate actively in making decisions right from the onset of patient care. The fast pace and the constant demand for rapid and clear thinking have always been attractive, as is the chance to be the first to see a patient, to gather all the relevant information, and then to ferret out the diagnosis. It is in the ED that I find a balanced mixture of the deliberative side of medicine with the more hands-on approach of surgery. But most of all, I enjoy relating to patients of different backgrounds and eagerly look forward to the opportunity to care for the great variety of patients seen in emergency and acute settings.

Example #3. The following personal statement offers an interesting combination of professional and personal reasons for selecting the specialty. However, the writer risks conveying the impression that he chose ophthalmology more as the result of a process of elimination than for its intrinsic attractiveness.

> Although I have long been interested in ophthalmology, my choice of the specialty was not an easy one. Only after sampling what many other specialties had to offer did I realize that none suited me as well. The chance to combine extensive patient contact in a clinical setting with the need for surgical precision, attention to minute detail, and aptitude in the most advanced technology medicine has to offer is an obvious attraction of the specialty. Of all of my clinical experiences as a medical student at UCSF, however, none rivaled the pure emotion I felt during my senior clerkship in ophthalmology, as I watched the vision of a patient with a dense cataract I had examined in clinic be transformed from mere detection of hand motion to near normal the next day as a result of the ophthalmologist's expertise.

[Long sentences.]

[Feelings seem disproportionate to event.]

Medicine as a Second Career

Example #1. In contrast to some second-career candidates, this applicant emphasizes the common ground between pediatrics and his previous career. In fact, the paragraph does not explain why he decided to make the career change.

> For five years prior to medical school, I taught computer science in grades 2–12 at a private bilingual school. I loved working with children and their families and had the joy of seeing my students learn and grow over a number of years. These same preferences led me to an interest in pediatrics as a specialty. Pediatrics is a heady mixture of the exotic and the mundane, of glowing health and desperate illness. It offers a wide variety of patients, a mix of common and uncommon disorders, a practice based in growth and development, and the possibility to make a real difference in the lives of patients and their families.

[Smooth transition.]

[Motherhood and apple pie.]

Example #2. Like many second-career applicants, this student also felt that something meaningful was missing from his career. However, he makes one misstep: In contrasting his future career in psychiatry with his past work in mathematics, he puts the latter down unnecessarily. While it is true that making a career change is not easy, characterizing a career change as a monumental achievement may sound overblown.

> My pure math activities were enjoyable for themselves, yet I had a growing sense that community service was what gave my life meaning and direction. Did I want to get to the end of my life and answer "What had I done?" with "I proved theorems"? Hoping to use science to help others rather than merely to create more science, I concluded I might be happiest in the long run in medicine, and courageously decided to change careers. So far, medicine has more than fulfilled my expectations as a context to combine the heart and the head. I am particularly intrigued by the doctor-patient relationship, which impresses me as a seamless blend of problem solving, hypothesis testing, trust building, and appreciation of the patients' individuality.

[Don't denigrate previous accomplishments.]

Example #3. This is a well-written paragraph that demonstrates remarkable insight and maturity of thought. The first half of the paragraph is a concise description of the applicant's activities during the year off. In the latter half, the applicant shares what he has learned without portraying it as an unprecedented revelation.

> After my third year of medical school, I pursued my interest in policy issues studying for a master's degree in public health at Emory. I spent the year exploring the epidemiology of infectious diseases, options for health care reform, and the empowerment of low-income communities. I learned useful skills in biostatistics and qualitative evaluation, and gained a global perspective on our health care system. At times, however, our discussions of abstract ideas and numbers felt too far removed from the realities of people's lives. I became convinced that debates about health care delivery should be rooted in concrete clinical practice, in the stories of patients and providers. My experience in public health taught me that doctors have a special role in society because they are trusted by patients and respected by policy makers. This combination allows physicians to be potent advocates for their patients and their community.

Good summary.

Nice tie-in with his interest in family practice. Clear, concise, and thoughtful.

Strong Extracurricular/Community Accomplishments

Example #1. This applicant has an impressive list of extracurricular activities and achievements. But it is the richness of detail that convinces you that she is diversified and involved in her community.

> Self-motivated, I work vigorously at my research, teaching, and patient care. However, it is also very important to me to continue furthering my personal interests, including the creative preparation and presentation of gourmet foods, wreath making, and horse training. Especially rewarding is my weekend volunteer work with the Stony Brook Riding Club for the Handicapped, which entails rounding up the herd at 6 a.m., feeding, grooming, tacking, and assisting the physically and/or mentally disabled riders in any way necessary. Annual CPR organization and instruction to the public brings important education to the community and keeps me abreast of the layman's current fund of medical knowledge. Additionally, my family background of being the eldest daughter of an architect and a nuclear medicine technologist from Indonesia has led me to a longtime interest in the integration of drawing and science, namely medical illustration. My aspiration is to obtain formal training in illustration technique when my medical education is complete; in the meantime, I hope to continue publishing my drawings and using them in presentations during my residency.

This sentence preempts any concern that the writer's extracurricular activities would interfere with her duties as a resident.

Be careful not to digress; they need a house officer, not an illustrator.

Example #2. It is not enough to list your academic accomplishments CV style. This student highlights the significance of his academic activities in clear, well-organized expository writing.

> Computer consulting work has provided me with close contact with creative researchers in science and medicine. A two-year thesis project with Dr. Elizabeth Rutter challenged my skills in relational databases, clinical record-keeping systems, and exploratory statistical techniques.

Emphasizes professional skills developed during the project.

> In the laboratory of Dr. Jeffrey Greenberg, I applied innovative real-time video microscopy and image processing techniques to fundamental growth and cell-division questions in cell biology. Through my lab work I have developed interests in improving the quality and utility of medical technology for clinical decision making.

Attempts to connect basic science to clinical research.

> I have supplemented medical school by being an active participant in basic biomedical science. In addition to medicine, I am familiar with the tools and vocabulary of modern molecular biology. I read a wide variety of clinical and scientific journals, and use literature searching extensively.

Applicant seeking a research-oriented residency skillfully weaves in additional academic activities.

Poor Academic Performance

Example #1. There is very little room for excuses in medicine. Either you got the job done or you didn't. Unless you have a glaring problem on your record, excuses will only cause the committee to focus on your weaknesses. In this example, the applicant tries to explain why he did not obtain more honors.

> On the wards, I found it easy to develop rapport with patients and team members. Ward medicine stimulated my love of scientific inquiry and problem solving. I found enthusiasm, dependability, focused presentations, and resilience keys to success. I excelled in medicine clerkships, but my other interests have often required making compromises in pursuing honors in all rotations.

Risky to make excuses.

Personal Experiences

Example #1. This applicant uses a barebones description of a patient experience to demonstrate her appreciation of the unparalleled access physicians have to their patients' intimate lives. A program director might not fully appreciate how a simple statement from a patient might affect a medical student.

> In my second year of medical school, I spent one afternoon each week with a primary care physician in San Francisco's Castro district. The practice specialized in caring for HIV-positive homosexual men. In addition to learning about the health care and social issues of this population,

Functional summary of volunteer experience.

> the patients and I grew comfortable with each other as I worked to earn their trust. The privilege of health care providers to share difficult times and confidential information with patients was clearly illustrated to me when after an interview a patient remarked, "You know, you're the only woman I've ever talked to about this."

Choice quote at end adds warmth.

Example #2. This applicant in family medicine makes a basic cultural and human observation through a touching yet humorous experience in an over-crowded Kenyan hospital. The richness of prose is matched by the complexity and maturity of thought underlying her observations.

> Note the lush and perhaps excessive detail.

I found the explanation for my surprising happiness one night in an unusual way. At 3 a.m. I was called to the wards to admit a young woman and arrived to find her comatose, moaning, and rocking on her half of a rickety cot. I examined her, hung IV quinine for likely cerebral malaria, did a lumbar puncture, and put down an NG tube as the entire ward of sick women gravely watched the proceedings, their faces eerily illuminated by my penlight, the only source of light. Last to do was the Foley catheter, but try as I might I could not locate the woman's urethra. One of the nurses began to giggle—just a little giggle. I began to giggle. The

> Very powerful.

women on the ward began to smile through their fevers, then chuckle. Soon the entire ward was laughing, great guffaws resounding through that miserable ward. I understood immediately. There was nothing vindictive or belittling in our laughter. On some unspoken group level, really a cultural level, we were pulling together to survive, transcending the almost unbearably hopeless human suffering. No one of us as an individual could hope to escape, but together, as a group, through this laughter—symbolic of some human universal, some common denominator—we stood a chance of retaining our dignity, our perspective, our

> Observations that bespeak intelligence and insight.

optimism. Thinking about this moment afterwards, and, indeed, about my whole experience at Mogashi Hospital, I have come to realize the crucial role that cultural constructs—shared belief systems, mutual ways of reacting to circumstances, family, friends, rituals, society—play in an individual's life.

Example #3. Anecdotes about patients are commonly used to highlight an applicant's compassion and sensitivity. Such accounts should, however, be used with discretion.

During the first week of my outpatient medicine clerkship I met Miss G., a 65-year-old woman who came to the clinic for a routine health assessment. During the course of her evaluation, I obtained a screening mammogram which unfortunately revealed a spiculated mass suggestive of malignancy. For the first time in her life, Miss G. faced the possibility of a diagnosis of cancer and realized she must come to terms with her

> Writer must have made a connection with the patient, but the message is not clear.

own mortality. For the first time in my life, I found myself looking into the eyes of a patient, trying to be honest and kind while conveying bad news. It was a moment I remember well. I saw Miss G. in clinic on several occasions over the ensuing weeks. Although she usually came to see me for health maintenance needs, we invariably turned to her concerns about breast cancer. She approached her fears with remarkable courage and stoicism, finally surrendering to tears of relief when her biopsy was found to be benign. I experienced both a sense of loss and a wonderful feeling of fulfillment when the months in the clinics came to an end. In

> Avoid criticizing "all my classes," as the reader probably teaches one.

retrospect, Miss G. taught me more about illness, therapy, and what makes a patient "feel better" than I had learned in all of my classes.

Strong Finishes

Example #1. This is an example of a strong finish, somewhat compromised by overuse of the first person singular. The applicant efficiently states his professional and personal goals, highlights notable personal qualities, and sets forth his expectations for residency training—all within five sentences. Unfortunately, each one starts with an "I."

> At UCSF I have experienced tremendous personal growth and have clarified my professional goals. I am committed to developing pragmatic multidisciplinary approaches to improving the quality and delivery of health care in the United States. Personally, I desire to provide compassionate and technically excellent medical care to patients from all walks of life. I will bring to residency energy, enthusiasm, integrity, and ability. I expect a challenging, rich environment in which to learn and practice good medicine.

Very concise.

Written with conviction and sincerity.

Example #2. Many applicants finish with a "ready for anything" type of statement without convincing the reader that they understand what they're getting themselves into. This applicant takes an honest look at the challenges ahead and her ability to meet them. In addition, she balances discussions of her career plans with a glimpse into her personal life. We see how the interplay between work and leisure maintains her balance and stamina.

> I know I have set high goals for myself: clinician, educator, and health advocate. The majority of the time I find working with underserved populations extremely rewarding; however, it can also be emotionally demanding. I have profound admiration for family physicians who have devoted their life to this work. I often grapple with the question of what will enable me to sustain this commitment for a lifetime. The combination of working at an individual level to address health needs and at a more macroscopic level to affect health policy is synergistic for me— each inspires my work in the other. On a personal level, I find my time away from medicine rejuvenating as well. Spending time backpacking, gardening, or being with friends and family enables me to return to work refreshed. Being a physician entails personal sacrifice and dedication, and I am eager to begin the challenge.

Dose of humility makes applicant seem more human.

Reality check shows forethought about career plans.

SAMPLE PERSONAL STATEMENTS

In the following pages, we have reproduced some successful personal statements in their entirety, edited only to protect the applicant's identity. Most of the applicants behind these statements matched at top institutions across the country. Once again, commentary is based on the observations of several residency directors, personal statement coaches, and a professional editor. Remember that your personal statement must reflect your own unique style and personality.

Personal Statement #1. The writer of the following statement left a career in neuroscience research to pursue pediatric neurology. Her statement effectively discusses her reasons for delaying medical school, disliking graduate training, and then ultimately entering medical school—thereby directly addressing the questions a director might have about an older applicant. The essay reads very naturally. Self-effacing humor and enthusiasm for the specialty inflect the essay and compensate for other shortcomings. The essay would have been improved, however, if the applicant had toned down her remarks about her love for the specialty.

Use the personal statement to tell your story. This is your chance to stand out from the crowd in a good way!

Good motivation.

Appropriate exploration of reasons for entering first career.

Dramatizes her shift in values.

Integrates awards into paragraph on interests.

When I first entered Oberlin College in 1980 I wanted to go into medicine—it took me 11 years to get there. When I first applied to medical school I thought about pediatric neurology—fortunately, it has not taken me another 11 years. During my third-year pediatrics clerkship, I told one of my best friends from college (who is now a primary care attending) that I absolutely loved going to work every day and that I was amazed at how much fun it was to "play with" your patients. Her response was that I could have children of my own and I didn't *need* to go into a field of medicine just to "play with kids." As I continued to love every minute of my other pediatric rotations, I began to realize that of course I didn't *need* to, but that I certainly *could* if it was what I enjoyed the most and what I seemed to do the best.

When I was in college, I initially put off medicine for entirely the wrong reasons: I hated the competition of the premeds, I could not imagine studying nonstop, and I did not want to stay up all night every three to four days for years of my life. Instead, I knew that I wanted to study the brain. I had two wonderful role models in my psychobiology career: I got my thesis published, and I headed to graduate school looking forward to a career in neuroscience research. But I feel fortunate now that my six years in a graduate program in experimental neuropsychology at UCSD showed me that a career in research by itself was not enough.

The turning point was deeply personal. My four-month-old niece was diagnosed with a grade 4 glioblastoma multiforme at the start of my fourth year. I remember sitting in the ICU waiting room at Denver Children's trying to concentrate on a paper related to my dissertation and realizing that what I was studying would never be directly helpful to this beautiful little child or to the rest of my family. It was then that I focused on why I had not been truly satisfied with my graduate experience—something was missing. And I came to realize that what was missing is the very thing that I need and want most from my career—direct application of my work. My personality needs more instant gratification than full-time research was bound to give me. In fact, the only gratification that I did seem to be getting routinely in graduate school was through teaching. I loved the interaction with students, the challenge of being an effective communicator, and the sense of responsibility toward the students, all of which are integral parts of being a successful teacher. I received the Distinguished Teacher Award in 1992 and was subsequently appointed to the teaching assistant consultant position responsible for training all the new TAs in the Psychology Department. Unfortunately, in much of academia, teaching is not as valued a commodity as it should be, and I was constantly made to feel that I was spending "too much time and effort" teaching. As for my research efforts, I am fortunate enough to have experienced the thrill that comes from finding the predicted effects during the final data analysis of my dissertation project, but I know that this thrill would have been magnified ten times if the research had been clinically applicable. I also realized that ultimately I wanted more out of my interaction with patients than having them as research subjects. My experience in medical school has taught me that I was right, there is nothing more rewarding than direct patient care—no matter how challenging it can be. The fact that a career in academic medicine combines the patient care, teaching, and clinical research that I value so much makes me realize how lucky I am to have found this path.

Despite the fact that it was a little disconcerting to turn 30 during my first year of medical school in a class whose mean age was 23, and that it may seem a little harder for me to stay up all night than for my 25-year-old classmates, I have never regretted my path. I feel that the life experience gained from my year as a social worker working with pregnant and parenting teens, and my years in graduate school have contributed immeasurably to my learning of medicine. I knew better during first and second year what was really important—not the grades that I received, but rather how well I could learn to apply that knowledge to a clinical setting. I can also look at the frustrated and angry parents of a sick child and understand a little better what they are going through by applying my experience with my sister and niece.

> Lighthearted acknowledgment that medicine is a second career.

> Demonstrates how maturity works in applicant's favor.

For a short time during my third year I allowed myself to be steered toward adult neurology by eminent senior faculty members, but I knew there was something in my heart that would not let me make a final career decision until I had experienced child neurology. I went into it with mixed feelings. Another friend who was finishing her pediatrics residency had told me that she had considered doing a neurology fellowship, but thought that it was "too depressing" . . . so she went into oncology instead. I must admit that this scared me. But I knew after only a few days that this was what I was meant to do. I enjoyed every patient interaction I had—the 14-year-old with a static encephalopathy and an intractable seizure disorder, the perfectly normal four-year-old who came for follow-up after a "bonk" on the head, and the eight-year-old with sudden onset of cranial nerve palsies of still unknown etiology. My learning curve was vertical and I went to sleep every night with Dr. Bruce Silverstein's text on my bed, and then was fortunate enough to have the opportunity to ask him questions in clinic in the morning. Many people have told me how lucky I am to have found a field that I am so enthusiastic about, that to fall so completely in love with something is what everybody hopes for. I knew that day that I went to Toys R Us (postcall) to buy a koosh ball to test visual fields and small plastic toys to test manual dexterity, and the night at 4 a.m. when I sat in a rocker to console a methadone baby in the nursery before going to bed for that all-important two hours' sleep, that they were right.

> Humor works surprisingly well here.

> You can chill; we know you like the specialty.

Personal Statement #2. The applicant has done a terrific job making her enthusiasm and convictions apparent to us. The introduction is unevenly written, but the decision to launch the essay with a set of reasons for specializing in pediatrics makes the essay focused and direct from the start. In the middle two paragraphs, the applicant's extensive community activities are well described. Overall, the essay is solid and persuasive.

Of the many contributing factors in my decision to pursue a career in pediatrics, the opportunity for patient education stands out as the most influential. During my clinical clerkships, I discovered many fields to be intriguing and learned from, as well as enjoyed, many aspects of each. It became clear, however, that the rotations providing more patient contact and continuity of care were the most fulfilling. My memories of third-year clerkships are of explaining cardiac catheterization to help allay fears, diagramming reasonable schedules of discharge medications,

> The writer scraps a superfluous introduction.

Good motivation.

Laying it on a bit thick with the community activities.

"Most rewarding experiences": Good way of organizing paragraph.

The writer describes a project from start to finish, showing that she can follow through.

and discussing puberty with girls beginning their development. Thus, choosing a field became not merely a determination of what I found to be intellectually challenging, but a selection of the role I wished to play in delivering health care to my patients. Pediatrics as a specialty allows the most interaction with patients and their families and affords perhaps the broadest role for the physician, including that of child advocate/social activist, health educator, family friend, and role model. Here, colleagues are interested in a patient's adoption history and school performance, and time can be scheduled solely for the purpose of STD teaching.

In my own educational experiences I have been blessed with supportive teachers who were also excellent role models. I was awarded the opportunity to enter a research laboratory as a high school student largely due to the commitment of a chemistry teacher and the generosity of a pharmacologist. This led to an aspiration to run my own laboratory with a program for future students. In college, a biochemistry professor's encouragement allowed me to pursue an individual project resulting in a publication. Perhaps as a means to reciprocate, I became involved in the local community. I performed the majority of my volunteer work through Alpha Phi Omega, a coeducational service fraternity affiliated with the Boy Scouts of America. Typical activities of the organization were Easter egg hunts for the county's foster children, creating a haunted house every Halloween at the Salvation Army, and providing aid in the aftermath of a local earthquake. Other community-oriented projects included tutoring of Chinatown youths on academic warning. As examples of Asians in college, the tutors also assumed roles of "big siblings" to help the students bridge cultural gaps and to encourage exploration of life opportunities outside the inner city. These activities eventually led me to realize that medicine, with its emphasis on service, would be the more satisfying career for me.

In medical school, I continued my community activities as time permitted. The two most rewarding experiences were that of teaching at a middle school and of organizing a series of talks for fellow pre-professional students. A few classmates and I taught middle schoolers through a program (Med Teach) coordinated by the medical school and the local school district. We had tremendous fun creating lesson plans for three classes each week, selecting different topics and styles of presentation for each age group. In addition to short traditional lectures, we often added interactive sessions such as class "Jeopardy" or "pin the organ on the body." One of our lessons on the eye even included group dissection of bovine eyeballs. This interest eventually grew to include the education of fellow classmates. As the community outreach chairperson for the Asian Health Caucus, I wanted medical professionals to learn about the special cultural as well as medical characteristics of the Asian patient (e.g., population differences in disease prevalence and drug tolerances). This idea of hosting a single lecture on an Asian health topic was discussed with friends, many of whom voiced wishes for similar talks on other cultural groups. Thus sprouted the day-long Multicultural Health Forum, which explored various cultures and their relevant health issues with speakers from different institutions. Moreover, I was able to secure sponsorship from the Department of Psychiatry and develop the forum as a credited class with availability to all preprofessional schools, including those of pharmacy, nursing, dentistry, and medicine.

I am eager to maintain my interest in teaching, both through patient education and through involvement with medical student training—

knowing well the difference an interested resident can make in the medical student experience. Because of this factor, there was never any doubt that I would be best suited for a university-based/affiliated pediatrics residency program. I currently anticipate a career in general pediatrics and therefore desire a well-rounded program with strong training in primary care. However, infectious disease and genetics are two areas which I wish to further explore with the option of possible advanced training.

Balanced and realistic discussion of career goals and training inspections.

Personal Statement #3. This applicant in plastic and reconstructive surgery does a particularly good job detailing research interests without overloading the reader. Note that he rarely has to discuss his interest in plastic surgery in abstract terms—specificity makes this essay work. Through careful attention to his prose, the applicant shows that he cares about his future career in plastics.

As a volunteer anatomy and pathology laboratory instructor, each year I am faced with a new set of students, unpredictable new group dynamics, and ultimately new challenges for presenting material. At times such as these, I truly appreciate the remarkable plasticity of the human mind. A principle taught to me by my college anatomy instructor, who influenced my career by teaching me *how to teach*, often comes to mind: "Answering a confused student's question with the same words repeatedly is like trying to cut paper by hitting it with a hammer over and over. Instead, trash the hammer and get a pair of scissors," she said, "or start tearing." Through the years, I have learned that effectual communication entails transmission of the understanding that you possess to others, so that they now also understand and are stimulated to think. This requires flexibility and patience, a good understanding and organization of the material, and a high degree of enthusiasm on the part of the teacher. While some of these attributes are inherent in my character, others have been learned and improved upon with every new enterprise.

Effective use of an anecdote to illustrate a point.

It is a similar challenge that attracts me to the field of plastic and reconstructive surgery, where often there are situations when operative procedures are modified to accommodate a patient's situation. Whether there is a paucity of soft tissue in one area, an abundance of skin in another, or a lack of bone due to destruction or congenital absence, the human body can be made plastic much like the mind modifying the procedures. I welcome and look forward to a lifetime career of meeting these types of challenges creatively in both the adult and pediatric populations, always keeping in mind aesthetics, prognosis, functionality, and the patient's wishes.

Interesting analogy—plasticity as a parallel between teaching and reconstructive surgery.

Creativity extends to the area of research, which, together with teaching, draws me toward a career in academics. To offer a patient an objective list of therapeutic alternatives requires an active hand in contributing to basic and clinical sciences while keeping abreast of the most recent advancements. As an undergraduate in kinesiology at the University of Miami Biomechanics Laboratory, I investigated the recruitment pattern of the medial and lateral gastrocnemius heads in the cat across a continuum of postural and movement demands. To further study pathophysiologic mechanisms of diseases in light of a surgical subspecialty, I completed a post-sophomore fellowship with the Florida State Department of Anatomic Pathology, gaining familiarity with frozen biopsy criteria and processing, histologic examination of surgical specimens, special stains, cytologic interpretation, and fresh anatomic dissection during autopsies. Interested in diseases of the musculoskeletal system, I researched a new monoclonal antibody, O13, directed against the p30/32 gene of Ewing's sarcoma and its cross-reactivities with other small round blue

Good use of specific details.

cell tumors. Possessing a special interest in pediatric orthopedics, I participated in many of the Toland Hospital for Crippled Children activities over the course of three years, including an anesthesia clerkship, contributing to research conducted in the Gait Laboratory, participating in rounds and conferences, and observing a variety of orthopedic surgeries, the majority involving congenital hand abnormalities. It was here that I met Dr. Kathryn Douglass of Baylor University, who introduced me to the notion of approaching a possible hand fellowship from the direction of plastic surgery. Now, with my current interest in plastic and reconstructive surgery, I am presently exploring with Dr. William Schrock at Baylor University the potential of capitalizing upon the angiogenic properties of fibroblast growth factor in the creation of flaps for larger wound coverage secondary to burns or other major trauma.

> The writer's name-dropping is effective because he substantiates the references and explains their significance.

Plasticity, also, is a key virtue during any residency. I am quick to learn new theories and techniques, and able to work well with a wide variety of patient and medical staff personalities. These attributes, coupled with patience and a good sense of humor, have been instrumental in my growth thus far and will continue to be the basic foundation of my philosophy for success in plastic and reconstructive surgery.

Personal Statement #4. This very capable statement shows a strong sense of purpose while reviewing several past accomplishments. It offers another example of how to make an applicant's interests appear coherent and consistent.

While growing up in Chicago, I was curious about the city's economic and social segregation, and what could be done to change it. As an English major at Ohio University, I originally intended to teach high school in the inner city, where I felt I might have an impact on education for disadvantaged students. During that time I founded one of the first inner-city Girl Scout troops in Akron and led a troop of 30 girls for four years. As the girls began to trust me, they started to ask questions about pregnancy, drugs, and STDs. Although I greatly enjoyed my role as an impromptu health educator, I sensed the futility of providing education without other health resources. Most of these girls received medical care for acute needs only; very few had access to regular primary care. I became increasingly aware of the need for partnership between health education and primary health care. My interest in these issues generated my desire for a career in medicine. I am particularly attracted to family practice because it integrates the roles of clinician, educator, and health advocate into the role of physician.

> Jumbled introduction; jumps from fact to fact too quickly.

During medical school my primary goal was to develop my clinical skills; however, it was important to me to continue to work with underserved populations to reaffirm my reason for studying medicine. After my first year, I received a scholarship from the Ohio Valley Homelessness Project to study health care access among homeless people. I became acutely aware of the impact of homelessness on health status, and this motivated me to involve other students in this issue. To this end, I helped found a free clinic for homeless people in the 2300 on Main homeless shelter. The Ohio University Students' Homeless Clinic is entirely run by students and volunteer physicians. Since 2001, over 200 students and 30 physicians have provided over 2500 patient visits free of charge. In conjunction with establishing the clinic, I also helped develop an elective, currently in its fourth year, on health issues among the homeless. I have remained extremely involved in running the homeless clinic since its inception and currently serve on the Board of Directors.

> Impressive achievement, described in detail.

In 2004, I received the Margaret Dawson Award for Outstanding Commitment to Social Action and Social Justice. This is the single award presented at graduation from the School of Public Health.

Working at the clinic constantly reminds me of both my powers and limitations as a future physician. Homeless people have myriad physical, social, and economic factors affecting their health; many have problems far too complex to resolve in a single visit. At first, I was frustrated if patients would come to the clinic requesting moisturizing cream or cough syrup, but were resistant to discussing what I deemed more serious problems—such as substance abuse or hypertension. Eventually, I learned that by first addressing the patient's presenting complaint we could establish trust, which might form the basis for a more continuous relationship. These long-term relationships are what I value most about being a physician. This was affirmed for me in my year-long longitudinal clinic at Swanson Hill Health Center in 2003 as well as during my current longitudinal clinic at the AGH Family Health Center. Through these experiences I have had the opportunity to work with patients on health-related behaviors such as smoking cessation. While trying to change behavior often seems futile or frustrating at a single visit, following patients over a year has shown me the value of incremental change toward healthier lifestyles. The challenges and the rewards of working in this setting reconfirmed my interest in family practice.

> Perceptive and succinct.

> Reinforces primary care philosophy.

Dealing with underserved patients' day-to-day medical needs stimulated my interest in studying health care policy on a more global level. As a result, I took a year off between my third and fourth years to pursue a master's degree in public health at Ohio University. My main focus was to examine the factors contributing to the shortage of primary care physicians in underserved communities. I became convinced that changes in medical education could have an impact on the number of primary care physicians in underserved areas. Along these lines, I was active on a student-faculty committee whose goal was to integrate more primary care and women's health instruction into the curriculum. In addition, through the Department of Family Practice, I am currently researching how medical students' experiences in the homeless clinic affect their choice of a career in primary care and their interest in working with underserved populations. When this work is complete, I intend to submit it for publication.

> The writer makes the year off seem a logical result of her passion for health care, not a deviation in any sense.

> Make sure your letter writer discusses any relevant research or extracurricular activity.

I know I have set high goals for myself: clinician, educator, and health advocate. The majority of the time I find working with underserved populations extremely rewarding; however, it can also be emotionally demanding. I have profound admiration for family physicians who have devoted their life to this work. I often grapple with the question of what will enable me to sustain this commitment for a lifetime. The combination of working at an individual level to address health needs and at a more macroscopic level to affect health policy is synergistic for me—each inspires my work in the other. On a personal level, I find my time away from medicine rejuvenating as well. Spending time backpacking, gardening, or being with friends and family enables me to return to work refreshed. Being a physician entails personal sacrifice and dedication, and I am eager to begin the challenge.

> Personalizes the statement.

The examples below can be used to see how some personal statements address issues particular to a specialty choice. Students usually use these statements to describe why they chose the particular specialty. You can see from the examples that there are many and varied reasons for students to become attracted to a particular career.

Anesthesiology

I have met each challenge in my life with hard work and dedication. Whether it was training for a marathon, working full time while going to school, or starting a family, I knew that by working hard I would succeed. That's why when I had to take time off during my undergraduate education due to the financial strains of living in New York and starting a family, I knew this would be a momentary delay in achieving my lifelong goal of becoming a doctor. After my wife and I were able to obtain some financial security, I finished my B.S. in physiology at the University of Arizona and was accepted into St. Lucas University School of Medicine.

St. Lucas University is located on the beautiful island of St. Kitts in the British West Indies. Most of the classes are taught by retired professors from U.S. medical schools. Besides the excellent education I received, the life experiences my wife and I gained living in a foreign country without the amenities of the United States were priceless. We will never forget washing our clothes in the sink or searching for propane gas to cook with on our stove.

I finished my basic sciences with a 3.96 GPA. I went on to score a 246/95 on the USMLE Step 1. My high score placed me at Douglas Medical Center (DMC) in Fresno, California, for all of my clinical rotations. DMC is an excellent county hospital affiliated with University Hospital School of Medicine, which accepts the best students from St. Lucas University into its clerkship program. DMC provided me with a well-rounded clinical experience and prepared me well for the USMLE Step 2, on which I scored a 255/98. Also, during my surgery core rotation my beautiful baby girl was born.

Although I have found all my clinical rotations interesting, I experienced the most excitement from my time in anesthesiology. Anesthesiology offers me the opportunity to integrate my basic science knowledge with clinical care. In no other rotation did I have the hands-on application of basic sciences; every OR case was a mini-experiment in pharmacology and physiology. The fast pace and the constant demand for rapid, clear thinking made my time in anesthesiology nothing but exhilarating. My rotation also showed me the various duties of anesthesiologists beyond the OR and the integral part they play in labor and delivery, the emergency room, the intensive care unit, and the management of pain.

On a personal level, I find my time away from medicine rejuvenating as well. Spending time running, mountain biking, surfing, and being with my wife and daughter enables me to return to work refreshed.

My career goal is to enter a university-based anesthesiology program. I believe my strong science knowledge base, clinical experience, and ability to make quick decisions are well suited for anesthesiology. I am highly detail-oriented and enjoy being part of a cohesive medical care team. I look forward to the education, practice, and research opportunities available in anesthesiology.

Dermatology

During medical school I became involved in research with Dr. Flynn in the Department of Anatomy and Neurobiology at Medical State University. I utilized the skills I had obtained through my bachelor's degree in visual arts toward our project. The manual dexterity I acquired through artwork allowed me ease in performing microscopic, stereotaxic surgeries; my work with chemistry in photographic development proved useful in immunohistochemical staining of our injection sites; and my illustrative abilities were applied in mapping the axonal projections of the nuclei. My background in art has provided me a breadth of knowledge that enriches my approach to medicine. I continue in my tradition of challenging myself in new areas: entering medicine with a background in art, presenting and publishing research, and now endeavoring to become a dermatologist.

Dermatology is the field in which many of my interests and skills converge. The pattern, texture, and color of artwork are discussed in a similar manner as skin pathology is described. I am confident in my ability to appreciate and interpret the visual manifestation of disease. I enjoy creating a precise image of primary and secondary lesions in order to develop a thorough and accurate differential diagnosis.

Comprehension of histopathology is essential to the study of dermatology. Through my prior work in a surgical pathology lab and experience performing biopsies in my dermatology rotations, I have acquired an appreciation of the processes involved in and the necessity of obtaining adequate samples of tissue for diagnosis and treatment. I have refined my procedural skills through my experience in microscopic surgery and in suturing Mohs repairs.

As with most areas of medicine, relating to patients with understanding and empathy is a priority in dermatology. I have developed my interpersonal skills by interacting with a variety of people through my study of art, my residence abroad within a different culture, and my current work in medicine. Open communication with others has come with ease. I value the mutual respect and trust that develops between physician and patient; I witness the healing effect that such a relationship has in treating patients.

As a field that continuously changes through medical and technological advances, dermatology encourages the ability to engage in research. Having completed a study observing trends in basal cell carcinoma in an individual surgery practice, I am currently coauthoring a chapter on different types of skin cancer, to be published in a medical journal designed for general practitioners. I anticipate continuing in research throughout residency and my career in academic dermatology.

One of my greatest motivations in studying medicine is the opportunity to study and learn throughout my career. My introduction to dermatology in medical school generated great interest and a desire to learn much more about its practice and new developments. I appreciate the expanse of material involved and knowledge yet to acquire in the study of dermatology.

Dermatology is a field in which I can continue to challenge myself. Through my rotations in surgery and general dermatology, I have discovered that it is the field of medicine to which I am best suited. I eagerly anticipate engaging in and contributing to the study of the skin and its manifestation of disease. My studies in art and involvement in research have enriched my medical education and will continue to provide a unique and enlightened approach to the practice of dermatology.

Emergency Medicine

During my junior year at UCLA, I became certified as an emergency medical technician (EMT), a decision that had a profound effect on my life. I was subsequently hired by UCLA Emergency Medical Services (EMS) and staffed the campus ambulance, serving as a first responder for all medical aid calls on the UCLA campus and neighboring communities. There was a tremendous sense of responsibility in being the first medical provider on scene to assess and provide treatment for potentially unstable patients in unpredictable environments. In addition to cementing my desire to attend medical school, my experience with UCLA EMS introduced me to the field of emergency medicine.

At the completion of my first year of medical school, I was awarded the Student Research Committee Fellowship. This fellowship supported a research project designed to evaluate the safety and efficacy of external cardiac pacing of patients with symptomatic bradycardia by paramedics in the prehospital setting. This two-and-a-half-year project was supervised by the medical director of the San Francisco Fire Department. The data demonstrated a trend toward increased survival among patients treated with external cardiac pacing compared to those treated with conventional therapy alone. Based upon this data, the State of California Emergency Medical Services Commission approved external cardiac pacing as first-line therapy for this patient population, permitting EMS providers throughout the state to perform this procedure.

Throughout medical school, I was aware of my interest in emergency medicine but made a conscious effort not to prematurely exclude other specialties. I thought I might find one clerkship to stand out among them all, calling me to devote my life to it. Instead, I found them all incredibly challenging and fulfilling, particularly those experiences requiring immediate decisions to be made, procedures to be performed, and, most of all, trips to the emergency department. My greatest sense of achievement, regardless of the clerkship, was when I was caring for patients with an acute illness, exacerbation of a chronic disease, or a traumatic injury.

I am eager to begin my residency training and look forward to expanding my knowledge base, becoming more adept in assessment, diagnosis, and treatment in the acute setting, and gaining the experience necessary to become a well-rounded, confident physician. I hope to train in a facility with a culturally diverse patient population and a broad variety of trauma, medical illness, pediatric emergency experience, EMS exposure, and clinical research opportunities. In addition to supporting my growth as a physician, I want to train at a program that supports my development outside the hospital, encouraging continued participation in my personal interests, such as exercising, camping, and traveling.

My long-term goals include attending in a high-acuity, academically oriented, Level 1 trauma center that conducts high-quality clinical research. I am also interested in pursuing a fellowship in emergency medical services to enhance my ability to promote quality prehospital care. My understanding of the field of emergency medicine has vastly matured from my days as an EMT. I now realize that the realm of the emergency physician extends well beyond the back of an ambulance or the entrance to a hospital. Emergency physicians are regularly faced with the entire spectrum of medical and surgical disease, requiring immense skill, diagnostic acumen, and empathy for both the frightened patient and concerned family members. In this era of managed care and cost containment, emergency physicians must be conservative in their diagnostic evaluations, yet remain aggressive in their pursuit of excluding acutely life-threatening illnesses. More importantly, emergency physicians serve as powerful patient advocates and valuable liaisons between the medical community and general public.

I feel I have proven myself capable of compassionate, competent care during my clinical years and have no doubt that I will greatly benefit from residency training in emergency medicine. I eagerly await the next phase of my education and welcome the challenges and excitement it will bring.

Family Practice

Although I started medical school with an inclination toward primary care, my choice of family medicine was not a foregone conclusion. I have considered many areas of specialty throughout my medical school experiences, but I keep returning to family medicine as the best match for my vocational goals and personality. Family medicine attracts me for several reasons. First, family medicine allows me to treat a wide variety of patient populations and illnesses. My medical school training and extracurricular interactions have given me the opportunity to serve all age groups, from infants to the elderly. I love children and gave serious thought to a career in pediatrics. Yet I also enjoy aspects of orthopedics, obstetrics, psychiatry, and geriatric care. I feel that family medicine offers me the most interesting spectrum of patient care. Although some may view this variety as a daunting challenge, I see it as a constant spark of excitement in the practice of medicine.

I also find family medicine attractive because of its role in small communities. Unlike other medical specialties, family medicine affords me the opportunity to live and serve in a small town. I feel that a family doctor can fill an important need in small and often underserved communities. I look forward to offering quality, up-to-date medical care in a setting where my patients and I interact on a first-name basis and where I can offer treatment based on perhaps a more intimate knowledge of my patients' backgrounds. I found this to be true during my family medicine clerkship in rural Idaho as a fourth-year medical student. My experience in Idaho convinced me that I could enjoy serving as a family doctor in a small community. On a more personal level, a small community is a great environment for raising a family, and my wife and I would like our children to grow up in such an environment.

I also feel that family medicine has a unique and vital role in educating families and providing preventative care. As I teach parents about developmental milestones and immunizations, give anticipatory guidance, and prescribe treatments for childhood illnesses, I do more than treat one sick child. As I teach adults principles of healthy diet and exercise, I do more than avert heart disease. Such education has the potential to help generations live healthy lives. Age-appropriate screening and counseling are other important roles I look forward to as a family doctor.

Several influential family practitioners in my life have given me additional impetus for choosing family medicine myself. Dr. Watrous not only brought me into the world, but he also delivered and continued to care for my twin brother and four other brothers and sisters over the years. Several years later, he was able to deliver my sister's children as well. Of course this scenario is not always possible in today's transient society, where people change insurance plans and doctors frequently. However, the opportunity for this kind of long-term interaction with families seems to still exist in instances in family medicine. As a teenager my family doctor became a trusted friend and respected adult figure in my life. Dr. Mathur was able to relate to my teenage issues and treated me with appropriate respect. He showed me that a doctor can have a positive influence on a patient's life far beyond traditional medical cures.

Years ago, I was stymied as I tried to select an undergraduate course of study that would best help me in a medical career. I consulted several medical professionals and asked their opinions as to which major would best help me in a medical practice. Many respected family practitioners advised me to major in business so that I could better manage my own family practice someday and assured me that such an education would benefit me in any type of practice. They also felt that choosing a major outside the basic science curriculum (which I would still be learning as a prerequisite for medical school) could only enrich and broaden my education. Now that I have decided upon family practice, I am grateful for their advice and look forward to applying some of the business fundamentals I learned in my own practice of medicine.

Finally, family practice appeals to me because of its focus on the family unit. My family—my beautiful wife and two children, as well as extended family—is the most important thing in my life. I want to become the type of doctor that my own children, wife, mother, and grandmother would feel comfortable and confident turning to for medical care.

"Far and away the best prize that life offers is the chance to work hard at work worth doing."
—*Theodore Roosevelt*

My parents carefully measured out their wisdom like coffee grounds: shake hands firmly . . . look everyone in the eyes . . . never complain . . . work harder . . . smile and enjoy . . . always do the right thing. The experience of living has been the water that percolates through these lessons, ultimately defining my cardinal principles of work and life.

Passion, beneficence, and excellence are fundamental to these principles and drive my pursuit of general surgery. Passion. Every day I strive to deserve the privilege of practicing surgery. From my earliest research experiences with cardiac surgery in dogs, I have aspired to learn enough, work enough, and care enough to earn the trust of my future patients and colleagues. This passion is my sustaining force. It is the excitement that kept me up through four emergency appendectomies starting at midnight. It is the calm that steadied my hand to insert a chest tube and drop a central line at a 4 a.m. trauma. It is the sympathy that gave me patience to hear Mr. H.'s story detailing each evening's mighty struggle to stuff a volleyball-sized hernia back into his abdomen for 22 years before coming in for surgery.

This passion motivates me to be a great surgeon. Beneficence. I am devoted to improving the way things work; I believe that basic scientific research and medical education are essential for enhanced patient care. However, administrative efforts outside the immediate realm of medicine are also important to forging advancements in health care. After identifying a deficit in funding of student research, I developed a proposal for an endowed fellowship for scientific investigation. Resulting from a combination of numerous meetings, letters, and a big piece of my heart, the alumni trustees, medical center administrators, and university financiers agreed to endow over half a million dollars for a fellowship to support medical student research. This fellowship is funded for perpetuity and provides $25,000 to one student annually to pursue independent research. The first fellowship was awarded this past spring to a promising second-year who wants to cure cancer. Whether or not she achieves her goal, it is the spirit and talent of thousands of students and scientists like her that impel progress in medical science. My desire and ability to produce tangible improvements will benefit the field of general surgery.

Excellence. I am always searching for ways to improve myself as a human being and as a surgeon. Because a problem-based curriculum afforded a flexible schedule, I was able to regularly participate in service projects, most often visiting elementary schools to discuss safe sex and drugs with high-risk children. Frequently, later in the evenings, I helped treat sexually transmitted diseases at an indigent clinic. I chose to explore fields related to a career in surgery through a year of independent research. By putting my head down to get through the daily grind, I overcame the obstacles of gel exposure snafus, cell culture contamination, and editing for publication, to be productive in basic and clinical projects. My achievements in this previously unfamiliar territory—I was a philosophy major in college—have given me the experience, confidence, and motivation to support research as I move on to my next stage of training.

This commitment to self-improvement maximizes my abilities and opportunities. By remaining true to my cardinal principles I will enthusiastically strive toward, and hopefully lead, the promotion of patient care as a surgeon. Benefiting from my experiences and equipped with knowledge, effort, and spirit, I am prepared to continue such work worth doing.

Internal Medicine

Choosing a specialty in medicine, like medical school in general, is a unique experience that will make a tremendous impact on the rest of your personal and professional life. Many students are dead set on specific careers before they even make their first shaky incision in gross anatomy. Others think they know which field they ultimately want to pursue, only to discover later on that everything about their chosen specialty disagrees with them. Then there are students like me, who go to medical school armed with the knowledge that ultimately they'll become doctors, but not really knowing which kind.

When I began my medical education, I was honestly surprised to learn that many of my new classmates were already committed to specific paths, some of them with extensive research and experience in their fields of choice. My older brother, who changed his mind at least three times before he applied for residency, had advised me to wait until the clinical years so that I could make an informed choice, and that had been my plan from the beginning. But as more and more of my friends began narrowing down their choices in the first two years of school, my plan to wait to make a decision suddenly felt like procrastination. Nevertheless, with limited clinical exposure and plenty of studying to keep me busy, I resigned myself to following my brother's advice and to wait until my third year.

Making the abrupt shift from bookworm to third-year clinical clerk was both a nerve-wracking and exciting prospect. Although we had discussed the doctor-patient relationship and the art of medicine during the first two years of school, the opportunities to practice those concepts were few and far between. Interviewing patients for an hour once a week didn't seem like a realistic picture of things to come (it wasn't). I was nervous about balancing a schedule that I knew would be hectic, being responsible for patients while trying to read about diagnosis, pathophysiology, and treatment. Mostly, I was excited that I'd finally have the chance to learn how to care for people and to explore possible future careers. My introduction to clinical medicine was cut short, though. That fall, my mother was scheduled for extensive spinal surgery in an effort to relieve years of discomfort, and I was granted a leave of absence by the school and returned to Los Angeles to be with her for the next six months. When I returned in the winter to begin my clerkships, I realized that it was impossible to finish all the necessary requirements in time to graduate in 1999, and I became a member of the class of 2000.

In retrospect, taking the extra time was a serendipitous blessing in disguise. It allowed me to objectively approach the clinical clerkships without rushing to make a career decision. As I rotated through the various specialties, I began to get a better understanding of what I found interesting. Initially, radiology was one field that intrigued me, combining technology and intuition to clarify disease pathology. I signed up for electives and became involved in research, hoping to further stoke my interest and solidify my desire to possibly pursue radiology as a career. Instead, it had the opposite effect. I quickly realized that although I found the images and technology amazing, I sorely missed the direct one-to-one patient contact that we had talked about during the first two years and that we had been introduced to during the third year.

People often say that the lessons learned along the way are what make a journey worthwhile, that the opportunities to gain insight and acquire knowledge can be easily missed if you simply focus on traveling from point A to point B. It is this idea that embodies my experiences in medical school and that has led me to my decision to pursue internal medicine as a career. What I've realized is that the things I find most rewarding are developing relationships with patients and being in an environment that fosters continuity of care. Caring for patients from admission to discharge and following up long term to provide for their health care needs is what I ultimately want to base my career as a physician upon. Everyone who goes to medical school has unique experiences that lead them to discover their own personal niches. To me, internal medicine covers a wide spectrum of disease pathology while allowing personal relationships to develop with patients, offering the ideal blend of academic challenge and personal fulfillment. In this way, I can share in the lessons learned from other people's journeys while I continue on my own.

Internal Medicine/Pediatrics

During a clerkship in my third year of medical school in my hometown of St. Louis, I was struck by a comment made by a nurse one morning before rounds. She recognized my name as being the same as two previous physicians who had cared for her and her family. These physicians were my grandfather and great-grandfather. She then went on to tell me that my great-grandfather had delivered her, and that my grandfather had cared for her during her childhood at his office. What moved me most about what she said was how tangible my relationship to my grandfather had become, and the very meaningful impact they had made on this nurse's life. I chose to go into medicine during college on my own accord, yet the fact that I have two previous family members who were a part of this profession gives me a profound sense of integrity and responsibility.

Throughout my schooling, working directly with people has always interested me. My experience while attending Loyola University in New Orleans, where I worked as a health assistant for two years, helped me realize that I would succeed in medicine. A month-long trip during my senior year of college to a village in Nicaragua challenged my ability to communicate and work with people, and solidified even more my desire to study medicine. Multiple involvements during medical school, such as coordinating a student-run clinic on several Saturdays, supported my interest in primary care and at the same time fostered leadership skills and a better sense of team spirit.

My rotation in internal medicine at a Veterans Administration hospital, the first of my third-year clerkships, initiated a desire to pursue the specialty of internal medicine. I was exposed to patients with conditions ranging from asthma to resistant HIV, which I found to be intellectually challenging and professionally fulfilling. Later in the course of my third year, my exposure to pediatrics paralleled my experience in internal medicine, and my learning curve took off even more. Now I find myself using the medical literature more frequently to support my rising interests. I find clinic to be a rewarding interaction and a wonderful chance to counsel parents/guardians. My interest in combined internal medicine and pediatrics as a specialty solidified at the end of my third year of medical school. Primary care is my interest. Seeing and helping patients of a wide age range and of various clinical presentations is what I want to focus on. My enthusiasm for internal medicine and pediatrics is both complementary and synergistic. I intend to take full advantage of the training offered and become an extremely competent, well-trained, and respected physician. In short, I want to be a resource for my patients and a source of appropriate medical care. The variety of patients in this setting draws me toward this field and will keep me continually interested and enthusiastic throughout the course of my career. The fact that I will comprehensively train in treating children and adults alike compels me to pursue internal medicine/pediatrics.

The bridge and relationship between the two areas, in my perception, are well connected. In my student experience, both internal medicine and pediatrics hold a common approach to patients. Their corresponding knowledge funds are both diverse and comprehensive. I look forward to being able to employ that knowledge competently and effectively throughout the course of my career.

Neurology

Among many other things I have learned in medical school, I have come to the opinion that the role people assume in the somewhat conservative field of medicine involves wearing a relatively thick professional mask. This is not necessarily negative, as there is no denying that an air of competence and compassion is certainly inspiring to patients. However, perhaps in part because I have never been a particularly accomplished actor myself, I find it all the more interesting when that mask is taken off and the true self emerges through all the layers of professionalism. When one truly enjoys his job, the most fun and energetic part of his personality emerges. When a patient presents with a rare and interesting disease, or when there is a captivating diagnostic problem, physicians who love their jobs bring their full intellect and attention to bear. Then, amazingly, all the layers of formality and pride are peeled away to reveal an enthusiasm to solve the problem and share their knowledge and excitement, which I find extremely infectious. In that moment when a diagnostic test is performed, or when a novel scientific result is on the brink of revealing itself, we are all transformed into a curious child all over again, whether we are students, attendings, or Nobel laureates.

I have chosen neurology as a specialty because it is a field that fascinates me to that point of enthusiasm—an enthusiasm that I wish to share with my patients, future colleagues, and students. I believe that the central nervous system has so much intrinsic interest that it draws a higher proportion of physicians who are genuinely captivated by their field. An important benefit from this is that it provides for the opportunity to work with others with similar enthusiasm, enabling a more enjoyable and educational experience. The clinical work is interesting and satisfying to me because of the close association of findings on the history and physical exam with the lesion location and etiology. I also find some of the more subtle cognitive deficits from brain pathology to be extremely interesting, shedding light on the function of arguably the most important, complex, and uniquely human organ of the body.

I feel that neurology remains a final frontier of biomedicine, with many clinical and scientific truths yet to be unraveled and translated for the benefit of human health and knowledge. In an era when molecular genetic approaches are rapidly revolutionizing the field of medicine, neurology stands poised to gain significant therapeutic benefit, as many cerebral disorders appear beyond our present ability to cure. It is especially fulfilling for me to be able to offer help in these areas where it is sorely needed, and I anticipate a day when we have the power to prevent or cure intractable diseases like ALS or Alzheimer's disease as research efforts from the Decade of the Brain yield fruit. During my third year of medical school, I had the exciting opportunity to work on a basic problem in neurophysiology at the National Institutes of Health with a fellowship from the Howard Hughes Medical Institute. From my experience at the NIH, I have gained an enormous appreciation for the scientific efforts in elucidating the workings of the nervous system and the process involved in finding treatments for specific disorders. I was able to meet very accomplished physicians in the research arena who serve as my role models. The experience has been instrumental in shaping my career aspirations to pursue a biomedical research career, which appeals to the creative side of my personality. In addition to medical and scientific impact, neurology and neuroscience are fields whose questions have far-reaching implications for apparently unrelated fields such as religion and philosophy. By providing insights into mechanisms of behavior and consciousness, it addresses critical questions related to our essential humanity, which I find extremely intellectually stimulating.

I hope that with my sincere passion for the field, a diligent work ethic, and a good-natured team attitude, I will be able to help alleviate suffering from neurologic disease and simultaneously learn about how our minds work. For the future, I hope to be a part of the forefront of our advancing understanding of the neurological sciences and use that knowledge to heal our patients and train others interested in the field. For these reasons, I have chosen to specialize in neurology with an eventual goal of practicing, teaching, and conducting research at an academic hospital.

Neurosurgery

Very few matriculating medical students can realistically determine their future career choices. We all enter with the altruistic goals of becoming caring physicians and making a significant contribution to medicine. As laypersons, we do not grasp the breadth of medicine and often are unaware of its specialization. I myself come from a medical family background and therefore had a somewhat greater exposure to medicine, but I was in no way qualified upon entering medical school to reach a conclusion regarding a career in a particular specialty. In spite of this, I always entertained the notion of becoming a neurosurgeon.

The central nervous system represented to me the most intriguing and complex human organ system. During my first two medical school years, I was fascinated by the study of the central nervous system, including its intricate three-dimensional anatomy, physiology, and pathology. During my third year of medical school, I gravitated toward the surgical specialties. I had the opportunity to become a member of the University of Mississippi neurosurgical team and participate in many neurosurgical procedures, an experience that I greatly enjoyed. The meticulous surgeries and the application of intricate anatomical knowledge and physiology markedly impressed me. Neurosurgery offers the challenge of not merely maintaining a patient's life, but sustaining their spirit, intelligence, and personality. Unlike almost any other field, neurosurgery deals with the elements that contribute to our consciousness and make us human. These experiences led to the coalescence of my decision to pursue a career in neurosurgery.

My professional goals include the completion of a comprehensive neurosurgical residency training in conjunction with basic science research experience and subsequently pursuing a career in academic neurosurgery. The academic discourse and the intellectual stimulation afforded in an academic environment are appealing as well as the opportunity to participate in the endeavor of furthering the scope of our knowledge. I will strive to follow the clinician/scientist model that I admire and hope to develop a research program complementary to my clinical interests. On my part, I bring the desire to work hard, participate actively in my own education, and make a positive contribution to my residency program and neurosurgery.

I believe that my credentials to pursue a career in neurosurgery include my strong academic background. I began my undergraduate education at Clemson University, where I was elected to the Phi Eta Sigma freshman honor society before transferring to Georgia Tech University because of my desire to be closer to my family secondary to an illness in the family. At Georgia Tech University, I was elected to the Phi Beta Kappa honor society and received the College of Liberal Arts and Sciences (CLAS) Outstanding Scholar Award, an award conferred on the graduating CLAS student with the highest grade point average. At the University of Mississippi School of Medicine, I was awarded the Board of Trustees Academic Scholarship and continued my strong academic performance. Additionally, I was honored with the Basic Science Research Scholarship on the basis of an original research proposal involving the synaptic integration and information processing carried out in a single nerve cell. The research culminated in a poster presentation at the Eastern Student Research Forum. I have used that experience to pursue neurosurgical research relating to spinal cord injury that is currently in progress.

Aside from academics, I have been active in the Mississippi Medical Association and have visited that state capital on several occasions to observe and participate in the lobbying process. Currently, I am serving on the Mississippi Medical Association's Public Relations Council and am participating in the planning of programs designed to increase membership in our professional medical associations and raise physician awareness concerning current medically related political issues in the rapidly changing managed care market. For recreation, I am an active participant in pickup basketball games and make an effort to weight lift on a consistent basis. I have also maintained an interest in the area of technology applications and recently published an article concerning the Internet's medical applications. I am also currently in the process of constructing a home page for the University of Mississippi's Neurosurgery Department.

Obstetrics and Gynecology

While my path to becoming a physician has always been a straight one, my interest in the field of obstetrics and gynecology has come full circle. During vacations from college, I worked in the office of an obstetrician-gynecologist in Washington, D.C. Excited by the breadth of patients that he saw, I was also impressed by the surgical nature of the field. Thus, I began medical school believing I would one day be an obstetrician-gynecologist. During my first two years of medical school, I drifted from this belief and considered the areas of medicine and pediatrics. However, the experiences of my third year helped me to better focus my interests. While I was impressed with the thought processes involved in the evaluation of patients during my medicine rotation, I was often frustrated by the inability to physically do something to help. During my pediatrics rotation, I was amazed by the young body's ability to heal, although I often felt this healing had less to do with the medical team than with the body's natural defenses. The resiliency of my patients, coupled with the opportunity to practice preventative medicine and primary care, initially left me thinking I would enter the field of pediatrics. I began obstetrics and gynecology excited to see babies delivered, but otherwise completely naïve that this was my calling. After just a short time on the rotation, I found myself feeling not obligated to read at home, but excited to learn more about the problems I had faced that day. As in pediatrics, it was refreshing to see a generally young, healthy patient population. However, unlike in pediatrics, in obstetrics and gynecology there was often the opportunity to physically do something that would lead to beneficial outcomes. I look forward to the opportunities to combine prevention and treatment strategies to keep my patients healthy.

I see my career occupied not just with medicine, but with health care policy and management. During medical school, I have come to appreciate the quantity and complexity of health care issues today. I realize that as a medical student and resident I must focus on learning the facts and skills needed to be a successful clinician, but I also believe that knowledge of and participation in the vast number of health care decisions being made each day is imperative for a clinician. For this reason, I plan to constantly continue my education, both in the professional setting and by earning a degree in either public policy or business administration. With knowledge and credentials, I will become actively involved in creating and implementing health care policy that focuses on the needs of patients rather than of insurance companies or administrators.

I have always had an interest in education and community outreach, and my goal is to make a difference in the policies of the health care system. Access to health care in rural and urban communities is a serious problem that our nation faces, and I feel obligated to use my knowledge and background to help, whether on a local or national level. My desire to improve communities in need is long-standing. An important influence on this interest began with my high school sociology teacher and friend, Mr. C. Progressive in his requirement of 20 community service hours per semester, he stressed the importance of reaching out to others. Because of his hands-on approach, I learned about my responsibility to help others.

Unfortunately, Mr. C. died of complications arising from AIDS in February 1994. At his memorial service, a speaker asked the mourners to look around the crowded auditorium full of people whose lives Mr. C. had touched, a group that represented just a fraction of the whole. The speaker reminded us that if each of us could touch just one other person in the same way, and that person would touch one more person, and so on, the memory of Mr. C. would never be lost. I choose medicine as my way to impart knowledge, to give hope, and to touch others with love and understanding.

Ophthalmology

A person who feels a specific calling in his life is a fortunate person. While we never know what the future may hold for us, having a definite direction in which to travel is a real blessing and a rare occurrence. My calling to pursue a career in ophthalmology came after three years of dedication to studying the human body, interacting with patients, and "trying on" various medical specialties in my third year of rotations. My interest in the eye, however, began in my second year, during the ophthalmology section of the mechanisms of disease class. I found the intricacy and vastly varied pathology of the visual system to be fascinating. Even more interesting was the small amount of clinical exposure to ophthalmology in our third-year curriculum. Except for four afternoons spent in ophthalmologists' clinic during the general practice clerkship, the eye was not discussed much, but I thirsted for more knowledge in this area.

My firsthand experience with ophthalmology came under the guidance of a second-year ophthalmology resident, whom I greatly respect spiritually, personally, and professionally. I met him at a church youth-group function, and he invited me to visit the triage area of the emergency department. I spent a day in the emergency room with him, where he showed me patient after patient, each case more interesting than the one before. The patients were very concerned about their vision. As he went through the general exam with me, pointing out the varying pathology, he calmed each patient by explaining the details of their illness and treatment. After watching him during a few more visits to the ER, I knew I wanted to be this type of physician. Furthermore, after a day in the OR with an attending physician and a few discussions with my student advisers, I knew I wanted to treat these types of patients.

During medical school, my family and friends, who remain a very important part of my life, complemented my influences in the medical field by providing support and fellowship in a nonacademic arena. My mother, a school psychologist, and my father, a retired USAF pilot, continue to provide counsel from my hometown in Florida. My brother, a lawyer (in a firm that represents doctors and hospitals), also encourages me from his home in Florida. Following their example, I have been able to establish a strong work ethic and moral basis from which to guide my career. I have also been fortunate enough to pass along my experiences and advice to the youth at my church during church functions, including the annual youth choir trip. Throughout medical school, I believe I have learned the value of hard work, punctuality, discipline, knowledge, and a good attitude. These values are contagious, and I look forward to bringing them to whatever work environment I encounter.

Ophthalmology contains all of what I love about the medical profession: medicine, surgery, treatment of both the old and the young, primary care, and specialized procedures. Ophthalmology is also a dynamic field, with frequent new advances in preserving or improving people's vision. I will enjoy the challenge of keeping up with new developments and will take satisfaction in contributing to that growth. Having a calling that will grant me the opportunity to positively impact people's eyesight and health while offering them compassion during a stressful time will be a rewarding experience and a rich personal blessing.

Orthopedic Surgery

Running has been an integral part of my life since high school, when I became involved in cross-country and track. During college and medical school I have continued running and have completed several road races and two triathlons. Running has taught me the value of patience, dedication, and perseverance; provided an outlet for stress; and kept me physically and mentally fit. It was also through running that I began to appreciate the importance of the musculoskeletal system. I would periodically sustain various sports-related injuries, which led to my first exposure to the field of orthopedic surgery.

While I believe the traits I developed as a runner prepared me for the rigors of surgery, my interest in orthopedic surgery stems from my fascination with the effects of structure on function. From fashioning various creations out of Legos as a child to constructing electronic circuits and building off-road remote control cars as an adolescent, I have always enjoyed learning about how things work. As a young teen, I built a cabin with my cousin and uncle. I was enthralled during each step of the process: drafting the plans, setting the foundation, constructing the walls, laying the roof, and weatherproofing the exterior.

The opportunity to visualize and mentally construct objects in three dimensions combined with an interest in how the building blocks of life are put together attracted me to organic chemistry and biochemistry. In these courses I learned how minor changes in molecular structure could have drastic effects on chemical properties. While exploring the structure and function of cells and molecules through research, I became increasingly fascinated with the anatomy and physiology of the human body. During medical school, I conducted research using a rat model to investigate the effects of interleukin-10 on inflammation associated with venous thrombosis. This experience allowed me to gain familiarity with operating on rats under a low-power microscope, examining and preparing surgical specimens, and taking gross and histologic photographs. I particularly enjoyed operating on the rats, which enhanced my interest in surgery.

In addition to acquiring new knowledge via research, I also enjoy sharing knowledge with others through teaching. My mentors demonstrated time and time again how the combination of hard work and talent could allow a person to reach his or her fullest potential. My father, one of my greatest mentors as well as a physician, has shown me that happiness and tremendous personal satisfaction can be acquired by making a difference in patients' lives. It is these principles as well as factual concepts that I strive to share with students. As a senior in college I helped other prospective medical students prepare for the MCAT by teaching classes for Kaplan Educational Centers. In the year before I began medical school, I was a teaching assistant for an honors organic chemistry laboratory and discussion group.

In medical school I have experienced tremendous personal growth and have focused my career objectives. Key elements that I have used to achieve continued success include maintaining a good sense of humor, learning how to work effectively with a variety of different patient and medical staff personalities, spending time with friends and family, and having interests outside of medicine. I will bring to my residency energy, enthusiasm, a strong work ethic, and a constant desire to learn new things and share ideas with others. I am seeking a challenging, engaging environment in which to learn and deliver high-quality care to patients. I hope to help myself and others fully develop our talents so that our patients can achieve optimal health, mobility, and function. I am looking forward to a challenging career in orthopedic surgery involving patient care, teaching, and future discovery.

I have always been driven by meeting new challenges, and it is that aspect of otolaryngology that is most attractive to me. The spectrum of ENT, ranging from microsurgical procedures of the ear to large head and neck cancer surgery, is one enjoyed by few medical specialties. ENT also encompasses allergy, infectious disease, and endocrinology, to name a few areas, and it is this broad scope of possibilities that has drawn me to the field. I am excited about working in a surgical specialty that gives me the opportunity to provide both primary and specialized care to patients of all ages.

I gained exposure to ENT during a surgical elective that was part of my third-year surgery clerkship. I had just completed my internal medicine rotation and was considering a career in medicine when I was introduced to otolaryngology. The ENT physicians I had the pleasure of working with demonstrated great knowledge of general medicine combined with excellent surgical skills. They had very good rapport with their patients, and they appeared to be some of the most satisfied physicians I had seen in my years as a medical student. They gave me hands-on experience in both the clinic and the operating room. By the end of my surgery rotation, I knew that I would be happiest pursuing ENT as my specialty.

I have worked hard during medical school to put myself in a position to be competitive for residency training in the specialty of my choice. I believe my work ethic stems from being raised on a dry-land cotton farm in West Texas. I was taught that people are judged by their integrity and their hard work, and any effort I made was expected to be the best I could muster. These values have served me well in all aspects of my life. They have provided me academic success at all levels, and they have been reflected in my clinical evaluations in each rotation. I also believe that my success in medical school is due in large part to my balance between my family and school. I am married to a terrific woman who has encouraged me at each turn, and I have a wonderful four-year-old daughter who keeps my world and priorities in perspective.

Outside of school and family, I enjoy golfing, hunting, fishing, and exercising. I have recently taken an interest in photography, and I plan to concentrate this hobby on wildlife and nature photography. My wife and I are expecting our second child, and we are all eagerly anticipating the arrival of the next addition to our family. This is an exciting, changing time in our lives, made all the more so by the prospect of a career in otolaryngology.

Pathology

"To Dr. Karen, with love, Timmy and family." This was the inscription on the inside cover of an 1899 edition of The Merck Manual that Timmy's mom gave me on the last day of my pediatrics rotation. At the bottom of the page, in royal blue marker, was the scribbled signature of a three-and-a-half-year-old, *"Tim."*

Timmy had mitochondrial encephalomyopathy. The clinical picture of his illness early on was that of failure to thrive, and he continued to have waxing and waning episodes of muscle weakness and neurological deficits, including a significant degree of hearing loss. He taught me to sign *"lion"* and *"tiger"* because these were two of his favorite stuffed animals; the reason he taught me to sign *"see ya later alligator"* is self-evident. He and his family struggled through several misdiagnoses, including cerebral palsy, until the presence of *"ragged red fibers"* on a muscle biopsy led to the correct diagnosis. I remember wondering at the time what ragged red fibers looked like under the microscope, and wishing that I could see them myself.

Then there was Chase. He was six months old, an ex-23-week preemie, third of triplets. He had spent all but four days of his life in the hospital, suffering from multiple complications stemming from his birth history and necrotizing enterocolitis in his perinatal period. His last night was also my last on call during my pediatrics rotation. I wept after watching my attending stand stoically with his hand on the shoulder of Chase's mother as she held her dying boy. The next day, after just 15 minutes of sleep, I was working in a primary care clinic that was about 25 miles away. I drove 70 miles an hour back to the hospital after receiving a call that the pathologist wanted me to attend the autopsy. Nothing unexpected was found on the gross, but I was strangely excited a few days later when the pathologist showed me the micro, which revealed gut bacteria in nearly every organ system.

Before entering medical school, I decided to be a pediatrician. As pathology continued to intrigue me during clinical rotations, I faced a dilemma. Pathology was exciting, interesting, and fun, but the lack of patient contact gave me serious doubts. Would I feel like less of a doctor if I never met another Timmy or held another Chase? I was born to blue-collar parents, grew up in a blue-collar neighborhood in Chicago, and had blue-collar friends. I wanted to make my parents—especially my father—feel proud. My mom trained my nephew to say *"Auntie Doctor"* any time he saw a woman with a stethoscope. Friends pledged to bring their sick children to me someday. Would they all be less proud of me if I never wrote a prescription, never again used my stethoscope, if they couldn't see that I too would help heal people because they didn't understand what I did?

So I delayed the decision. I started my fourth year still answering *"I'm not sure"* to questions about my specialty choice. Then I began a pathology elective and sought the advice of my attendings. They were offended when I asked questions like *"Were you ever disappointed that you won't ever make anyone better?"* They reminded me that their work makes a difference every time one of them calls the results of a frozen section back to the OR, or determines whether a lesion was merely dysplasia or carcinoma in situ, or looks at a bone marrow to see if chemotherapy has been effective. I was ashamed at having asked the question.

It is possible that no one will ever again call me *"Dr. Karen."* It is probable that I will never again receive a gift from a patient. And I am not holding my breath for Christmas cards. But I will make patients better. I will make a difference in their lives by giving them the peace of mind of knowing what caused their loved one's death, or perhaps by finding what everyone else missed to provide a diagnosis. I will be excited and challenged and I will have fun as a pathologist. Whether or not my dad will ever understand what ragged red fibers are remains to be seen.

When I was in kindergarten and got asked the question "What do you want to be when you grow up?" there were really only two acceptable answers. I could choose a life of either fighting crime as a policeman or extinguishing blazing infernos as a fireman. I chose fireman. As I got older, the same question became more difficult to answer because the choices became more varied and the decision held more gravity. The question wasn't so simple to answer anymore. I went through third-year rotations in a quandary about this decision when it suddenly became so simple: I want to do something where I wake up in the morning and can't wait to get to work, and at the end of the day I am sad to leave. This is pediatrics for me. Some say that children are just little half-sized adults, but I choose to differ. They are their own individuals. Children possess an honesty about them that adults have lost somewhere along the way, and they will openly share with you this honesty. I still remember Maria, the two-year-old with acute gastroenteritis who hugged me and planted on my cheek the biggest, wettest kiss I have ever had the pleasure to receive. She was convinced I was the one who had made her feel better. Of course there was also Mikey, a four-year-old with a sprained wrist who was very verbally profound in how much distaste he had toward me after I attempted to manipulate the wounded wrist. Then there are the difficult cases that eternally remain etched in your brain. Karen, an eight-year-old with eczema herpeticum that had spread to cover both eyes and eventually sealed both her eyes shut. It is experiences like these that can cause a person to hesitantly leave the floor at the end of a hectic day and want to come back in the morning hopeful to see what a new day has in store.

Several other experiences also shaped my decision to enter into pediatrics and work with children. During my undergraduate years at a large public university, I was involved in a study of methylphenidate in children with attention deficit disorder. Being a psychology major, I found the research extremely intriguing and found myself enjoying spending time with the "difficult" children. While in medical school I worked with the Department of Child and Adolescent Psychiatry at Westchester Medical Center developing an alternative method of therapy for reaching children and adolescents diagnosed with a history of both substance abuse and physical abuse. This was based on previous studies, which demonstrated that traditional "talk" therapies are not as effective for children who have suffered severe emotional distress. For these types of patients, other modalities of creative expression had to be developed. This proved to be one of the most challenging yet rewarding projects I ever had the opportunity to be involved in.

For my current project, I have chosen to explore a different venue in child care. I am currently in the process of compiling the research for my master's thesis in public health. I chose to pursue a joint MD/MPH degree after being inspired by other physicians with MPH degrees that I worked with at the National Institutes of Health. My thesis centers on the topic of pediatric emergency room utilization in a metropolitan area. I hope to provide evidence of incorrect utilization of the emergency room for nonemergent health issues and underutilization of the primary care physician for these nonemergent situations. In addition, I will attempt to establish that incorrect utilization of the emergency room may have indirectly contributed to the rising cost of health care. In the future, I plan to use my MPH as a tool to create positive changes not only in ER pediatrics but also in the field of pediatrics in general. Whether it is in the area of maternal-child health or even policy for prevention of pediatric disease, my goal is to make a difference in the realm of child health care.

So what do I want to be when I grow up? I want to be challenged every single day of my life. I want to feel the satisfaction that what I do improves the lives of children in big and small ways. Most importantly, I want to be enamored by the work I do . . . I want to be a pediatrician.

Physical Medicine and Rehabilitation

"A very good one!" That's the way I answer people when they ask me what kind of doctor I am going to be. This has been my answer since I started medical school. Growing up in a family of six, with two educators as parents, I was taught to strive for excellence in whatever I do. Although the start of my medical career was somewhat turbulent, over the last two years I have demonstrated this attribute in all of my medical school activities. I must say that taking a leave of absence from my medical education was one of the best things I could have done. It enabled me to refocus my life and rededicate myself to medicine. Never has my determination to become a physician been stronger.

I have chosen to pursue a career in physical medicine and rehabilitation for three main reasons. First, I am intrigued by the area of study. Throughout my medical education, I have been very interested in neuromuscular medicine. I can remember back to anatomy lab, when I was amazed at the way our neurological system was "wired" to the rest of our bodies. Never during my basic science education was I more curious; an elective rotation in PM&R solidified this interest even more. I look forward to the challenges of treating patients in this field.

The multidisciplinary approach to patient care is another reason I like PM&R; I have always felt that the team approach to almost anything was the best way to go about things. I see myself as a "team player." My interpersonal skills are very good, and my abilities to lead a group have been demonstrated as the director of a summer camp. Sitting in on "team rounds," I found a great sense of accomplishment in seeing that all of these people were working toward a common cause. I can see how the ultimate goal of helping the patient is better met in this setting.

The last reason I have chosen PM&R as a specialty is my appreciation of the way that this field approaches the patient. I have always felt that patients should be seen as individuals, not cases. I have found that PM&R, unlike most other fields, pays very close attention to the psychosocial aspects of medicine. Patients are seen as mothers, husbands, students, and workers, etc. I feel that this is the only way to truly deal with the care of patients. It is relatively easy to "treat" a disease, but only through a holistic approach can one hope to "heal" a patient. As a candidate for residencies, I feel that I possess traits that many programs are seeking: enthusiasm, a strong work ethic, and a positive attitude. I have often been told that the vigor with which I approach life is contagious, and that my upbeat attitude is appreciated by many of the patients I have seen. I work hard at whatever I am doing yet have the ability to put life into perspective. I believe that these aspects of my personality will make me an asset to any residency program.

In summary, I am an enthusiastic, hard-working individual with a positive attitude who is dedicated to the field of physical medicine and rehabilitation. I hope that I will be given the chance to elaborate these thoughts in an interview with your program.

Psychiatry

The story is told of the late Wilfred Bion that another analyst once consulted with him regarding the case of a schizophrenic who would wake up in the middle of the night to see if he was really there. Bion thought for a moment and then commented, "Well, everyone deserves a second opinion." Indeed, when I informed my family and friends of my choice to go into psychiatry, I found myself with more "second opinions" than I had ever bargained for. One resident told me he was surprised, since he thought I was very motivated and interested in medicine. Other medical students commented enthusiastically that they admired me for choosing such a difficult field. Invariably, this was followed by a story about a person they had heard about who had left surgery—or obstetrics, or medicine—to become a psychiatry resident, after a psychotic episode in which he or she had almost killed several patients. Strangely enough, no one could tell me which program the resident was in. My interest in psychiatry comes from several different perspectives, which is probably why I find the various biological, social, and psychodynamic aspects of psychiatry so interesting. As a psychology major at Princeton, my courses were mainly biologically and pharmacologically oriented. I wrote my sophomore and junior papers on the psychobiology of seasonal affective disorder (SAD), and then spent two summers in Oxford studying the epidemiology of SAD. Yet, driven by a deeper desire to be able to understand and communicate with as many people as I could, I also studied three different languages at Princeton, was a peer counselor, and sang with three choruses. After college, I taught mentally retarded and emotionally disturbed adolescents, where I learned how to talk to and work with children who had problems ranging from autism to severe hyperactivity, and also spent much of my free time in the deaf community, where I learned about cultural values and the responses to societal pressures in closed communities.

Upon my arrival at medical school, I didn't know if I would go into psychiatry. I was fascinated with how the human body worked, and thought that the cerebral challenge of diagnosing physical disease might be more compelling than the gentle and creative exploration toward understanding the origins of a woman's depression or personality disorder. However, my unconscious betrayed me—I spent much of the time with my medical inpatients talking about what their illnesses meant to them or how their families dealt with their hospitalization. Throughout my third year, I found myself sitting with patients like the young woman at the OB/GYN clinic who admitted with shame that she was being hit by her boyfriend; a gigantic nightclub bouncer at the ambulatory clinic complaining of fatigue, who was just starting to adjust to regular life again after being in jail for 11 years; and a middle-aged woman with unexplained chest pain in the ICU, who cried and held my hand as she told me about months of insomnia and sadness following her painful divorce. I knew this was what I wanted to do.

As for the future, I still love research and will be doing a few months of research this year on the topic of memory in survivors of childhood trauma, but I also have a strong leaning toward psychotherapy and am giving serious consideration to becoming trained as a psychoanalyst. Eventually, I would like to have a career in an academic setting, where I can focus on patient care using both psychodynamic and psychopharmacologic techniques, and also teach and do some writing or research. Yet, wherever my future lies in these changing times, I know that as long as I have the unique opportunity and privilege to sit with people, listen to them, and help them tell their stories, I will always be satisfied.

Radiation Oncology

My decision to become a physician was influenced by several factors that led me to pursue a career in an oncologic subspecialty. My grandmother was diagnosed with breast cancer that later metastasized. My grandfather was diagnosed with lung cancer after having smoked for over 30 years. Recently, my cousin was diagnosed with melanoma, which later spread throughout his body. He was treated with advanced oncologic treatment, including radiation therapy, before passing away a few months ago. These experiences, along with a family friend who is a radiation oncologist, solidified my goals to become a radiation oncologist. Helping my family has given me an understanding and sensitivity for treating cancer patients.

Before learning about cancer through firsthand experience, I worked with cancer patients while volunteering at local hospitals while at the university. Volunteering was invaluable because the patients were very eager to share their experiences with me. I was fascinated in biochemistry classes and research by the interactions of genes, normal and mutated, that lead to neoplastic growth.

While working toward my MD degree at the State University of Medicine, my interests were again fueled by classes and conferences concerning oncology. I started my third year with a surgical oncology rotation under Dr. Johnson and Dr. Smith, who challenged me and taught me the surgical aspects of treatment. Dr. Galvez, my preceptor for gynecologic oncology, allowed me to participate in Tumor Board conferences. These increased my awareness of the risks and benefits of the numerous gynecologic treatment modalities.

Radiation therapy engages my interest because of the chance to cure and offer palliation in a minimally invasive to noninvasive manner. I am gratified to be involved in a treatment modality that offers relatively immediate and anatomically directed results. I am amazed by the wide spectrum of clinical cases one sees as a radiation oncologist. I also saw patients treated for heterotrophic bone growth and management of cardiac transplant rejection. Through research, I am involved in two projects at S. Cancer Center with the Radiation Oncology Department. One project entails biliary duct carcinoma and the other involves spinal cord carcinomas and gliomas. I am also comfortable offering palliation to terminally ill patients because I know that advances will shift to an increasing improvement in treatment and hopefully cure.

I have discovered many things about myself. Clinically, I can easily establish rapport with my patients. My evaluations consistently commend my ability to form strong patient-physician relationships. If I do not know the answer to a patient's question, taking the time to learn from and consult with an attending or resident allows me to answer the patient. There is no greater tool for learning than teaching someone else, and in that light I hope to remain in an academic setting as my career progresses. I am a diligent worker and an excellent time manager. I will happily spend extra time with a patient because as Dr. Khan, my preceptor in radiation oncology, says, "When I am with you, YOU are my only patient."

During my residency I wish to obtain excellent clinical and academic training that will provide a strong foundation for a successful and fulfilling career in both an academic and community setting. A quote I found in a book reminds me of the difference I hope to make in people's lives:

"A hundred years from now it will not matter what my bank account was, the sort of house I lived in, or the car I drove . . . but the world may be different because I was important in the life of a patient."

Radiology

Sure I will become a doctor. But what field of medicine will I choose? To find the answer to this ever-present question, I entered my clinical clerkships with an open mind, looking to discover my strengths and interests. As I went through my third-year clerkships I saw appeal in each experience; however, as the year came to a close I still had not found a niche. I began to look beyond the core clerkships I took as a third-year student. The vast number of career options for aspiring physicians can be quite overwhelming. So I decided to persevere in the manner in which I undertake most tasks. I stood back and thought, evaluating positives and negatives, and evaluating myself. I realized that perhaps the best fit for me was possibly something that I had exposure to during every third-year clerkship, yet its intricacies and true definition were still very foreign. This field was radiology.

Radiology can easily be taken for granted by an inexperienced medical student such as myself. It is ingrained in our heads that to rule in or rule out certain diagnoses on our differential often requires a visual study. The patient goes off to another place and receives this visual study, and soon thereafter a report is made revealing the medical situation that is occurring beyond the human eye. What this place is like and what the people do there began to capture my interest. It seemed quite ideal for a person such as myself who found interest in each clerkship I was exposed to during my third year. It allowed diagnosis in the medically ill, in the young child and infant, in the psychiatric patient with mental status changes that cannot be ruled out by history and physical alone—and of course it allowed diagnosis in the surgical candidate. Radiology in a sense allows exposure to the entire potpourri of medical specialties, therefore allowing continuing diversity but from a specialized viewpoint.

Realizing the specialty that appeals to you is one step; deciding whether you feel you can succeed and contribute in that area is the second. As an incoming resident I feel I have many attributes that suit me to be successful in radiology. First, I feel that the old adage that all radiologists sit in a dark room away from all other human contacts is incorrect. Interpersonal skills are essential for a successful radiologist. Patient contact does occur, although on a limited basis, and interaction with other physicians, whether as a consult or as a fellow radiologist, occurs on a daily basis. I enjoy interacting with others and feel my personal skills will provide a comfortable environment for patients and colleagues. Second, I enjoy variety but at the same time realize that I prefer to focus within a specialty. I enjoy anatomy and anatomic relationships, which is also applicable in the field of radiology. Third, I have come to learn that I am quite visual both in my approach to learning and in my everyday tasks. The field of radiology allows me to take advantage of this ability. I have also always enjoyed solving mind puzzles and games. Radiology allows me to take these visual puzzles, if you will, and put the pieces together to make a differential.

A career in radiology provides the challenges and intellectual interests that I desire in my chosen field of medicine. I feel that by not making a career choice until after evaluating every clinical experience with an open mind, I have made the correct decision. Given the opportunity, I feel I have the abilities and determination to succeed and develop into a competent radiologist. My success throughout medical school helps to demonstrate my drive and self-motivation. I have confidence in my abilities, enjoy working as a member of a team, and feel I can be a strong advocate for my patients. With my skills and motivation I feel I will be a valuable member to the field of radiology.

Urology

I performed my first surgery at the age of 12 during a Boy Scout campout. My surgical staff, the other members of Troop 148, watched around the operating/picnic table as my attempts to clean the only fish caught that day developed into an exploration of fish anatomy. I was fascinated by the intricate anatomy of living things. I eventually realized that surgery was not only an exploration but also a chance to heal.

During my high school years, my mother was diagnosed with a rare cancer of the kidney. Despite a nephrectomy and short periods of hope, the cancer eventually metastasized to her liver. Surgery was no longer an option for her, and she began a difficult path of chemotherapy. She died a few years later, but her death did not dim my surgical aspirations. Rather, it made me determined to become a surgeon who strives to improve surgical treatments while maintaining empathy for the suffering of my patients. My research, teaching, and clinical experiences have strengthened this resolve and have helped me choose urology as my future career.

My research experience began during my undergraduate education. Intrigued by the challenges and complexities of basic science research, I continued my research endeavors during my first and second years of medical school. I worked with Dr. Durbin investigating the use of antigen cytokine fusion proteins as a means of achieving antigen-specific alterations of the immune response. I also participated in clinical research during my final two years of medical school. I worked with Dr. Perry on a retrospective study to evaluate the utility of preoperative CT scan in staging patients with colon cancer. I enjoyed the intellectual challenge of laboratory and clinical research and realized its potential to improve patient care. The field of urology is rich in research opportunities, and I look forward to continued involvement in research both in residency and beyond.

I was given unique teaching opportunities in medical school, being selected as a teaching assistant for human anatomy and as a USMLE review course instructor. As an anatomy teaching assistant, I led daily small group discussions and cadaveric dissections. I gained a deeper appreciation of the complexity and variability of the human body while increasing my communication and teaching skills. I enjoy teaching and helping my peers learn. I look forward to the opportunity to both teach and learn from my patients and colleagues as an academic urologist.

My clinical rotations were especially influential in my decision to become a urologist. I enjoyed all of my clinical rotations and hoped to find a surgical specialty that would offer a similar diversity of clinical experiences. To me, urology provides an ideal blend of surgical precision and medical management and a wide spectrum of patients and problems. In the future, I would like to specialize in one of the many available subspecialties in urology. I am especially interested in urologic oncology.

Surgery, whether on a picnic table or in a sterile room, still inspires me as it did as a child. My research, teaching, and clinical experiences in medical school have been instrumental in focusing that interest to the surgical specialty of urology. My knowledge has grown since my first fish surgery, but I still feel the awe at the complexity of anatomy and how much more there is to learn. I look forward to the ongoing opportunities to learn and contribute as I strive to advance treatment and patient care within the field of urology.

NOTES

Gearing Up for Interviews

You can breathe a small sigh of relief when invitations for interviews start coming in. You have cleared the first major hurdle in the match process, and your foot is in the door of several programs. Now, however, you need to maneuver the rest of yourself through the doorway.

HOW DO I PREPARE FOR THE INTERVIEW?

Good preparation for interviews is essential to making the best impression. Being overtired, disorganized, inappropriately dressed, or upset about travel glitches can only hurt your chances. In this chapter, we will walk you through the stages of interview preparation.

Scheduling Interviews

Many program directors will tell you that the date of your interview should not make a difference. However, conventional wisdom favors choosing the latter half of the interview season so that committee members will better recall your application during ranking sessions.

For many applicants, the crucial interview period begins after Christmas. For this reason, last-minute scheduling changes are very difficult to make during the peak interview months of January and February. Travel to the Northeast is especially unpredictable. The blizzard of 1999 and, more recently, the bitter cold of January 2003 forced thousands of applicants to cancel or reschedule key interviews. If you are in an early Match, you will be interviewing from September through December. Remember, if you want maximal flexibility in interview planning, you **must** turn in your Electronic Residency Application Service (ERAS) application or paper applications early.

If you get your ERAS application in early, you will likely be invited to interview early as well. Most programs have an administrative assistant who is in charge of scheduling. He or she will e-mail you a list of available interview dates from which you can choose. At this point in the program, you will have to sit down with a calendar and draw up a few possible scenarios in order to maximize the efficacy of your interview trip and prevent overcrowding of your interview schedule. Doing this will also allow you to save a bit of money in what can be a rather expensive process.

Schedule the most competitive and your most desirable programs in the middle of your interview schedule.

The interview process can be more grueling than you think. So for starters, **don't schedule interviews too close together.** Instead, space interviews at least two days apart so that you'll have time to travel, recuperate, and digest information from the previous interview. You should also schedule the most competitive and desirable programs in the middle of your interview schedule. By then you should have reached peak interview form without having lost your enthusiasm and energy (see Figure 10-1). In fact, many applicants end up canceling interviews near the end of the season out of apathy and fatigue. If you decide that you do not want to make an interview appointment or cannot do so, inform the program as far in advance as you can so that they can fill your interview slot with another applicant. Although this is a matter of simple courtesy, remember that reports of bad manners travel far in the small circle of residency program directors.

You should also try to arrange interviews in geographical clusters so that you can easily drive between sites or take advantage of cheaper regional travel options (see "Planes, Trains, and Automobiles" below). It is not inappropriate to politely request an interview at a specific program if you will be traveling to that general area for other interviews. Ask if rounds or a morning conference is a scheduled part of the day's activities. If not, ask if you can attend one or the other as part of the interview day. Rounds/conferences are often one of the easiest and most useful ways to judge the style and caliber of a program.

Mock Interviews

When you hit the interview trail, you want to be in fine shape. Real interviews are time-consuming and take serious effort to set up. You should also remember **never** to treat a real interview as a practice session even if it is at one of your less desirable programs. You never know how a visit might affect your rank-order list, especially if you end up bumping one of your lower-ranked choices to the top of your "most wanted" list.

Set up a mock interview early.

After four years in medical school, however, anyone can lose their interviewing finesse. So to get a little practice before the real thing, set up a mock interview early in the fall with your career adviser or another faculty member in the department. Ideally, this person should be an active member of the selection committee in your specialty. However, if you are interested in remaining at your home institution, be cautious! This information may be used when you are discussed during intern selection. Before you go in for your mock interview, review Chapter 11. Then have your "interviewer" conduct a "tough" interview with hard questions, especially if he or she has a reputation as a "softy." These tough conditions will give you the confidence you need to get through a hard interview when the time comes. Afterward, your "interviewer" should give you detailed feedback on the ease/confidence with which you handled the questions, the quality of your answers, and other personal characteristics that you projected during the interview (e.g., maturity, thoughtfulness, intelligence, ability to think quickly).

Tough mock interviews will prepare you for the worst-case scenario.

It is especially important that your interviewer be critical of your performance and your ability to maintain a conversation. You should ask him or her how you can ask more questions of the interviewer, as the most successful inter-

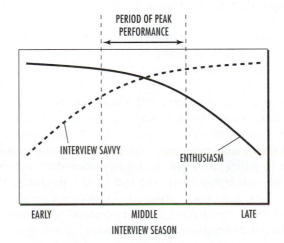

FIGURE 10-1. Performance during interview season.

201

viewers tend to do the least amount of talking. In general, the more someone gets to talk about himself or herself, the happier they will be with the conversation.

Finally, do not get overwhelmed by negative feedback from this mock interviewer. If you have a nasty habit of interrupting someone midsentence, it is better to know now and to keep it in the back of your mind when the real interviewer walks into the room.

If you want to squeeze even more feedback out of your ersatz interview, you can have it videotaped or audiotaped and then review it with your "interviewer." Try to evaluate yourself from his or her perspective. You can also simulate other aspects of the interview by coming to the "office" in full interview dress, carrying a folder of materials, and forcing yourself to stew a few minutes outside with the secretary because the interviewer is currently with another applicant. In a similar manner, you can assemble as complete an application file as possible, ask your "interviewer" to review it, and have him or her ask you questions based on your file. For the truly obsessive-compulsive, there are interview coaches who can play the interviewer, videotape the session, and coach you to a fine-tuned performance.

Doing Your Homework for the Road

One week before an actual interview, call the institution to confirm the date, time, location, and interviewers. If you have any of your interviewers' names, try to build on this knowledge. Is your interviewer a researcher, a clinician, a house officer, or an administrator? Once you've found out this basic information, get to work. First, call up local contacts (e.g., graduates from your school who are currently in the program) or ask the program's administrative assistant about the interviewer's specialty, personality, etc. Find out where they attended medical school and completed residency, as they may know people at your home institution. Second, run a MEDLINE search on the interviewer(s) and read their abstracts. Try to discover mutual interests to use as potential topics for discussion during your interview. You should also Google the interviewer's name. Finally, check out the program's departmental Web site (if applicable) to learn more about the faculty and program. Your goal here is not to appear political or "calculated" but rather to be prepared to highlight any strengths you have that might appeal to the interviewer. Even if what you learn does not come up in conversation, you will gain a psychological advantage just from knowing something about the interviewer. Remember, he or she already knows a great deal about you, so doing your homework offers you a chance to level the playing field a bit.

Level the interview playing field by learning about your interviewers.

In preparation for the interview, you will want to organize the information you have obtained about each program (see Figure 10-2). To do so, place all the material you have gathered in a labeled folder. If you have time, review this material and **jot down questions and concerns** that come to mind for that program. Interviewers will expect you to know about their program and to ask questions. This demonstrates a true interest in the program. You should also create a folder of your own application materials (see Figure 10-3). Of course, residency directors will also have this information—plus your application—in front of them when they interview you, all of which is fair game.

☐ The *First Aid for the® Match* Program Evaluation Worksheet
☐ The full FREIDA printout
☐ Informational brochures and pamphlets
☐ A photocopy of your application
☐ Any notes that you picked up from faculty house staff or fellow students
☐ For the research oriented, a MEDLINE search of your interviewers' publications
☐ A color photograph of yourself if one was not sent to the program
☐ Information from the program's departmental Web site
☐ Printout of program Web site

FIGURE 10-2. **Checklist for program information.**

Interview Attire and Grooming

First impressions are important. Even before you smile and say hello, your interviewers are evaluating what they see. So remember: Do not dress for where you are; dress for where you want to be. Then look at yourself in a full-length mirror. What do you see? Is the person staring back at you businesslike and polished? If not, you may want to reassess your choices. Also try asking someone whose opinion you value about your appearance. Does he or she agree with your assessment? Remember, too, to check the weather projection for the city you are visiting and dress appropriately. Most interviews occur in late fall and winter, so dress for warmth and comfort. Clothes are not the only factor, however; proper grooming is essential. Your overall impression will be enhanced by a recent trim or haircut, proper nail care, and very light if any perfume or aftershave.

Many programs will offer coffee, lunch, or snacks throughout the day, so consider having breath mints accessible. Do not use chewing gum as an alternative. Choose meals wisely, as stains at lunch remain present during afternoon interviews.

Just for men. Attire for men is rather straightforward: business suit, tie, and dress shoes. There is no one right color for a suit, but once you have chosen your color, remember that your shoes, tie, and shirt must coordinate. The most popular colors for suits are black, charcoal, and blue. Black, charcoal, and navy suits look best with black shoes. Dark brown suits look better with dark brown shoes. Speaking of shoes, shine them.

You never get a second chance to make a first impression. Now is the time to splurge on quality interview attire.

☐ The dean's letter
☐ Copies of any letters of recommendation that were made available to you
☐ Copies of your transcript(s)
☐ Your CV
☐ Your personal statement (especially if you personalized your statement)
☐ Reprints of any noteworthy publications
☐ A copy of your *First Aid for the® Match* worksheet of application requirements (Appendix B)

FIGURE 10-3. **Checklist for folder of application materials.**

203

Professional alterations are a must if you are an "off size."

Avoid lethal doses of aftershave or perfume on interview day.

A man can say a lot with his choice of tie. For instance, a tie with cartoon characters may be great for a party, but a solid or simply patterned tie is best for interviewing. A white or ivory shirt in a good fabric will complete the look. If in doubt, choose a white shirt. Remember, however, that while a white shirt is a good choice, white socks are not. Choose socks that match or are darker than your pants or shoes. Jewelry is another aspect of attire. A watch—preferably a dress watch—is acceptable. Earrings and visible body piercing are not. Light aftershave or none at all is best.

Two suits should suffice for the interview season. Alterations are a must if you are not a standard size. Each suit may be used for two to three interviews if no spots or spills occur. Have your suits dry-cleaned during a break in the interview schedule. Pack a portable iron and a lint brush for trips, and inspect your suit closely before packing to ensure that no spots, lint, loose threads, or holes are present.

Just for women. The motto for women should be "professional yet simple." This is the time to splurge on clothing. A well-made, classically cut suit will serve you well. For the conservatives, it is still more acceptable for women to wear skirts. However, increasing numbers of women are also choosing pantsuits. You need to be comfortable in your interview day clothing. If you will be uncomfortable in a skirt, a tailored pantsuit and a confident attitude may serve you better. If you opt for the traditional skirt suit, remember to choose the right length for your body style. The length of your skirt should be no shorter than the top of the knee and no longer than two inches below the knee. This is largely an issue of practicality, as a skirt that is too short will show too much leg when you are sitting, while a skirt that is too long will hamper mobility when you are walking. You should also wear stockings. Choose something close to your skin tone in a color that complements your suit. Well-made stockings have a finished appearance. Always pack an extra pair of stockings, as finding a hole or a run in a stocking on the morning of an interview can be a disaster.

You may need two solid-colored suits depending on the number and timing of your interviews. Wool and cotton-blend fabrics travel best and wrinkle least. Linen wrinkles easily and is not warm, so it is probably not a good choice. Women tend to know what color looks best on them. On the interview trail, basic black, navy, and dark gray are the most popular. Classic colors such as evergreen, dark brown, or maroon can serve as alternatives.

The blouse is next to the face and neck, so choose a color that complements your skin tone. You can wear something other than white or ivory. A patterned blouse is acceptable if properly chosen. A conservatively cut blouse made of silk or linen fabric looks professional yet feminine. Shoes should be sensible yet stylish. Low-heeled pumps that complement your suit are most comfortable for walking and appear professional. Jewelry is an accessory that should not detract from your finished appearance; simple studs, small hoops, or pearl earrings work well with most suits. Depending on the blouse, a strand of pearls or a simple chain is optional. A dress watch and a simple ring are also acceptable. Multiple earrings and visible body piercings are not. Inspect your appearance once your outfit is complete.

If you choose to wear makeup, use it to enhance your appearance. Remember that less is more. A light coverage of foundation, blush, eye color, and mascara can complete the picture without adding distraction. A matte lipstick of coral, light pink, or brown will complement your outfit without appearing obvious.

If possible, do not carry a handbag. A leather attaché case or satchel is a better alternative and can accommodate paper, pens, keys, makeup, and comb or brush.

Unfortunately, interviews will cost most of you a lot of time and money. During the 1999–2000 interview season, students reported spending an average of 20 days away from medical school at their program interviews and paid $2000 for application fees and travel expenses (see Figures 10-4 and 10-5). Plan to spend more money and more time away from school if you are applying in a competitive specialty.

In most cases, it is possible to make travel arrangements for your interviews without razing your bank account. To some extent, the most cost-efficient means of transportation depends on your geographical location. Some parts of the United States have better rail service than others. In some areas, a rented car may be your best option. The next section will introduce you to some ways to minimize your travel expenses.

Planes, Trains, and Automobiles

American Airlines Meeting Saver Fares for the AAMC Student Residency Interview Program. Discounts of 5% off the lowest coach fare on American Airlines fares are available only to senior students in AAMC member institutions during the interview season through this program with the Association of American Medical Colleges (AAMC). For more information, call:

American Airlines Meeting Services Desk
(800) 433-1790 and reference the AAMC index #17603

If you have any questions, contact Denine Hales, dhales@aamc.org.

Discount regional airlines. In light of recent competition from low-fare airlines such as Southwest, you can obtain very reasonable airfares when traveling regionally (see Table 10-1). As with other airlines, tickets are cheapest with a 21-day advance purchase and a Saturday night stay. With discount airlines, you may encounter less choice in flight times and more stopovers.

Southwest Airlines (800-I-FLY-SWA, www.iflyswa.com) is a regional airline that has grown rapidly since its inception in 1971 and is now the fifth largest

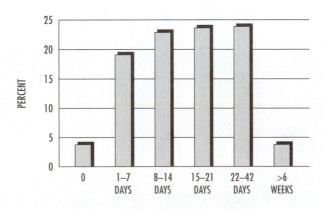

FIGURE 10-4. Days spent interviewing away from school.

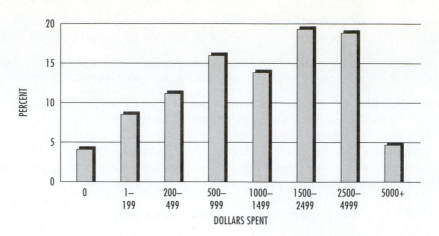

FIGURE 10-5. Amount in U.S. dollars spent applying and interviewing for residency positions.

Some airlines will charge a service fee for booking over the phone, so buy your tickets online if posssible.

airline in the United States. Southwest takes pride in its low fares and customer service, and its Web site is extremely user friendly. Another perk is Southwest's cancellation policy. If your plans change and you need to cancel or reschedule, you can apply the original purchase price of your travel toward future bookings (within one year) without penalty. Other airlines charge $100 or more in penalties for canceled reservations. (See Web site or contact a Southwest agent for details.)

Low-cost airlines. These upstart airlines (see Table 10-1) generally provide a price break when compared to the major airlines. Often, however, they will not appear in travel agents' computers or on some Web sites, so you may need to go to each airline's Web page directly.

Amtrak. Amtrak offers deals on multi-ride tickets for short distance travel within the Northeast, Midwest, West, and South. The California Rail Pass offers seven days of travel in a 21-day period for $159. One year of unlimited travel in Florida is $249 with Student Advantage ($20 annual fee, www.studentadvantage.com, 877-2-JOIN-SA) and AAA members are eligible for discounts. See the Amtrak Web site for weekly specials and advertised specials. For more information, call or visit:

> Amtrak
> (800) USA-RAIL [(800) 872-7245]
> www.amtrak.com

Metro-North Railroad. Because the entire Eastern seaboard is well connected with light rail, rail is a viable alternative to driving, especially given distances of 200 miles or greater. Reasonable fares are available even with little or no advance reservation. To receive general rail schedules for the New York metropolitan area and Connecticut, call:

> Metro-North Railroad
> (800) METROINFO
> www.mta.nyc.ny.us/mnr

In general, rail travel may be a more useful throwback than you think; you can use the time to review interview materials, rest, or catch up on other reading, none of which is possible when you drive. It's also harder to get lost!

206

TABLE 10-1. Discount and Regional Airlines

AIRLINE	PHONE NUMBER	WEB SITE
AirTran Airways	(800) AIR-TRAN (800) 247-8726	www.airtran.com
Alaska Airlines/Horizon Air	(800) 252-7522	www.alaskair.com
America West Airlines/ U.S. Airways	(800) 327-7810	www.americawest.com www.usairways.com
American Trans Air (ATA)	(800) I-FLY-ATA (800) 535-9282	www.ata.com
Frontier Airlines	(800) 432-1FLY (800) 432-1359	www.frontierairlines.com
Jet Blue	(800) JET-BLUE (800) 538-2583	www.jetblue.com
Southwest Airlines	(800) I-FLY-SWA (800) 435-9792	www.southwest.com
Spirit Airlines	(800) 772-7177	www.spiritair.com
Sun Country Airlines	(800) 359-6786	www.suncountry.com
Ted (part of United Airlines)	(800) CALL-TED (800) 225-5833	www.flyted.com

Travel agencies. You can purchase a ticket directly through the airlines described earlier, or you can visit your local travel agency. One student-oriented discount travel agency is STA Travel at (800) 781-4040 or visit www.statravel.com. Travel agents have access to information about the lowest available airfares on all major airlines. Unfortunately, however, some discount airlines, such as Southwest, are not listed on their computers. Travel agents' services are free to you, since their commissions are paid by the airlines. In general, try to purchase tickets three weeks in advance for the cheapest fares. You should also make sure that the airport you fly into is the best one in terms of price and distance from your program destination. You must balance the airfare with the time and cost of a taxi or shuttle to your lodging.

Internet travel agencies have proliferated because of their usability and cheap prices. Listed below are some of the more popular sites.

- **Priceline** (www.priceline.com). Priceline's Web site allows you to search for affordable fares or to name your own price for your airfare. After you enter in your desired travel plans, Priceline will search for any airline with the lowest fares, similar to other Internet travel sites. You can then select the carrier and flight times best suited to your needs. Priceline also offers

"Name Your Own Price," which can often yield a better deal. You choose your desired airport, the amount you wish to pay, and your credit card number. If an available fare matches your criteria, your card is charged. Once you have purchased your ticket, you cannot change, transfer, or cancel it. You should also be aware that although you choose your travel dates with the "Name Your Own Price" option, the airline will choose the travel times (which will range between 6 a.m. and 10 p.m.). Priceline will search for nonstop flights first, but there is a chance that you will have to make a stop or a connection.

- **Cheap Tickets** (www.cheaptickets.com). Cheap Tickets has been providing discount airfares on major airlines since 1986. To use it, you will need to establish a free profile. After you have done so, finding fares is easy; the site will lead you through a series of drop boxes. Using your search parameters, the site will list available flights from which you can form an itinerary. When your search results are shown, you will be told what the lowest available fare is, but you won't be told if a seat is available. You will then need to click on the "Seat Availability" button. Remember, however, that the available seats may not be at the lowest fare. If you did not get a seat at the lowest fare available, click on the "Fare Rules" button to view the restrictions for the lowest fare. You can then try to make modifications to your flight parameters in order to receive the low fare. A Visa, MasterCard, or American Express credit card can be used to purchase flights. Cheap Tickets charges a processing fee per order. Be sure to check their "Specials" page as well as their hotel discount and rental car pages.
- **Expedia** (www.expedia.com). Expedia has a variety of features you can use to check for airfares. You do not need to be a registered member to use the various search engines, but you will have to establish a free member profile if you wish to purchase a ticket. Expedia's basic fare search is similar to that of other Web sites in that it will search for the lowest airfare once you have typed in your search parameters. Expedia allows you to reserve your flight itinerary until midnight of the following day, but the fare is not guaranteed. Other search options include "Fare Compare," which will list flights similar to yours that other Expedia.com members have found. There is also the "Flight Price Matcher," which employs the same concept as Priceline.com. With this feature, you get to pick the price you are willing to pay for your flight. If a match is made, your credit card will be charged immediately. Some hints for getting your fare are as follows: (1) travel on a Tuesday, Wednesday, or Saturday; (2) plan a Saturday night stay-over; and (3) be flexible about your travel times and connecting flights. As with other sites, Expedia.com has hotel discount and rental car pages.
- **Orbitz** (www.orbitz.com). This is another Web-based service that surveys multiple carriers. Note that not all fares are available through Expedia or Orbitz, so be sure to check more than one source. Orbitz also offers hotel and rental car reservations.
- **Travelocity** (www.travelocity.com). Travelocity has the basic airfare, hotel, and rental car search engines. It also has a "Fare Watcher" feature that allows you to pick certain cities for which the Web site will continually check for low fares. You will need to register before you can use any of Travelocity's features.
- **Lowest Fare** (www.lowestfare.com). This site allows you to check airfares and seat availability without having to register first. (Of course, you will have to register to purchase tickets.) Be sure to check their specials, which are on their home page. Lowestfare.com also gives you access to maps and weather information in a selected city.

- **Kayak** (www.kayak.com). Many airline and hotel Web sites offer exclusive deals or low fare guarantees. Kayak allows you to search most of the sites for the best deals. You then book directly with the airline or hotel Web site to avoid fees charged by travel agency Web sites.

Where to Stay

You will need to take overnight housing into account as part of your travel plans. It isn't always necessary to figure big bucks into your budget for this item, so consider the following possibilities:

Free or low-cost accommodations arranged by the program. Some programs—especially primary care programs in the Midwest and East—will provide complimentary or discounted lodging at a nearby hotel or guest house. If your program does not volunteer information about such arrangements, ask the administrative assistant if any are available. You might also consider asking the residency program about staying in the residents' call room if one is available. However, be sure to find out if this room will remain unoccupied during the night so that you will be able to sleep well. Not only will this room be free, but you won't have to worry about finding your way to the hospital on the morning of the interview!

For women: AMWA Bed and Breakfast Program. The American Medical Women's Association (AMWA) has a "Bed and Breakfast Program" for members traveling to residency interviews. A member calls AMWA and specifies her destination. AMWA then supplies her with a list of members in the area, mostly physicians who have agreed to provide short-term (one to three days') lodging for other members. The student is then responsible for making arrangements with the host. There is an administrative fee of $10 for students and $15 for physicians. To use the service or for more information, contact Mare Glanz at:

Lodging can cost you more than airfare, so plan ahead.

> American Medical Women's Association
> 801 North Fairfax Street, Suite 400
> Alexandria, VA 22314
> (703) 838-0500
> www.amwa-doc.org
> E-mail: mglanz@amwa-doc.org

Recent graduates from your school. Some student affairs offices maintain lists of recent graduates and their residency programs. Not only are recent graduates at your target programs an invaluable source of information about the program, but they might offer to put you up for a night when you visit.

Other applicants. On the interview trail, you often meet applicants from the schools and institutions you will later be visiting. They may be friendly enough to offer you housing when you visit their home institution or just show you around the evening before the interview. If they will also be visiting your school at some point, consider extending them the same courtesies.

Accommodations recommended by the program. If you are stumped for housing options or prefer more luxurious surroundings, you can always check out local hotels recommended by the program. Residency programs often make arrangements with a hotel to offer discounts if you mention that you are interviewing with them. This information is frequently included with written invitations for interviews. If you don't get the official word, you can ask the administrative assistant for suggestions.

Hostels lack amenities like ironing boards.

Hostels. Hostels are cheaper than hotels because you will be sharing living quarters with your fellow travelers. Bathrooms and living rooms are communal, and sleeping quarters usually consist of a dormitory-type setting with bunk beds. Hostels are a great idea if you are staying in a city for more than one night, because you will be able to meet others who are interested in exploring the area. You should, however, try to find out as much information as possible about the hostel, including the location (is it near noisy nightclubs?) and general atmosphere (party crowd versus quiet folks). If you are a light sleeper, consider the fact that you will be sleeping in the same room as other people who may snore or come in late. Also ask if travelers are required to complete chores as part of their stay. Hostels are generally safe, but be sure to keep your valuables with you or locked up in the hostel's lockers or safes. Remember that not all hostels take reservations, so have a backup plan. For more information, check out the following resources:

- *Hostelling U.S.A.: The Official Guide to Hostels in the United States of America*, Washington, D.C.: Hostelling International, 1995.
- Hostels.com.
- Hostelling International (www.iyhf.org).

Budget-priced chains. Finally, you can simply go with a budget hotel/motel chain. If the residency program is not helpful with names and numbers of nearby lodging, you can call any of these major chains (see Table 10-2). Many have a AAA discount. When you make your reservation, ask about the room. Common concerns include a nonsmoking room, location in a quiet part of the hotel/motel, and a phone connection. And for security, is there a deadbolt lock? A peephole in the door?

University dorms. Many residency programs are located at colleges and universities that rent out empty dormitory rooms for $15 to $30 per night. Unfortunately, programs sometimes neglect to mention such accommodations in their brochures.

Handy Travel Tips

Arrive early; leave late.

Print your boarding pass off the airline's Web site the night before to save time.

Finally, we offer a few additional pointers to make your interview trip as smooth as possible:

1. Plan to arrive at your accommodations no later than the afternoon of the day before your interview. This will give you a chance to get oriented, adjust to time-zone differences, and handle any unexpected mishaps (e.g., lost luggage). If you are planning to fly out the day of the interview, check with the departmental secretary to make sure there are no further events scheduled for later that day. About departures: In general, it is better to leave later in the day so that you can have extra time to talk to house staff and faculty or to see more of the hospital and facilities.

2. When flying, try to take everything as carry-ons. You can bypass the crowded airport counter for a gate check-in and eliminate the chance that the airline will lose your luggage. We suggest a durable garment bag or a roll-aboard suit carrier for your interview clothing. If you must travel

TABLE 10-2. Major Budget Hotel/Motel Chains

HOTEL CHAIN	NUMBER	WEB SITE
Baymont Inns	(800) 4-BUDGET	www.baymontinns.com
Club House Inns	(800) CLUB-INN	www.clubhouseinn.com
Comfort Inns	(800) 4-CHOICE	www.comfortinn.com
Country Inns and Suites	(800) 456-4000	www.countryinns.com
Courtyard Marriott	(800) 321-2211	www.courtyard.com
Days Inns	(800) 325-2525	www.daysinn.com
Econo Lodge	(800) 4-CHOICE	www.hotelchoice.com
Fairfield Inn	(800) 228-2800	www.marriotthotels.com
Hampton Inn	(800) HAMPTON	www.hampton-inn.com
HoJo Inn	(800) 654-2000	www.hojo.com
Holiday Inn Express	(800) HOLIDAY	www.ichotelsgroup.com
La Quinta Inns	(800) 531-5900	www.laquinta.com
Motel 6	(800) 4-MOTEL6	www.motel6.com
Ramada Ltd.	(800) 2-RAMADA	www.ramada.com
Red Roof Inns	(800) THE-ROOF	www.redroof.com
Rodeway Inns	(800) 4-CHOICE	www.rodeway.com
Super8	(800) 800-8000	www.super8.com
Travelodge	(800) 255-3050	www.travelodge.com

heavy, at least pack your interview essentials (e.g., program interview materials, application materials, and interview suit) in a carry-on.

3. Pick up an updated discount travel guide. A particularly useful book (it saved one of us, stranded at La Guardia, several hundred dollars on airfare) is *Travel Smarts: Getting the Most for Your Travel Dollar* (Globe Pequot Press) by Herbert Teison and Nancy Dunnan. This guide, or a similar book by Consumer Reports, will stretch your travel dollar and minimize traveling hassles without sacrificing comfort.

4. If you plan on driving to most of your destinations, get a good U.S. map/road atlas for trip planning. Carry a pocket local map for each city you visit, or tear out the detail pages from an inexpensive road atlas. If you belong to the American Automobile Association (AAA), call or visit your

Give yourself plenty of time to get through increased airport security.

local office once you know your itinerary. Membership privileges usually include free road maps and customized routing advice. It's also worth inquiring about discounts on car rentals and lodging; many AAA clubs offer coupons for these services. And if you should have car problems en route, an AAA card can often save you much more than the cost of the annual membership fee. Before you set off, have your car properly winterized and tuned; ask the service station attendant to check your fluids and tire pressure and to replace your windshield wipers if necessary. Be sure to keep your car registration, inspection and insurance papers, and auto club materials in the glove compartment. If you don't already have one for your car, buy a flashlight and batteries—particularly if you will be driving at night.

5. If you have the time, the interview season can be a great way to mix business and pleasure. You can squeeze in some sightseeing if you have more than a day between interviews. That way, you'll get to unwind between interviews and learn more about the local attractions in the vicinity of the program.

6. Be sure to check local weather conditions in the city where you will be interviewing before you set off. This is especially important if you are traveling to an unfamiliar part of the country or if you are flying to a region with an extreme climate.

References

AirTran Airways Web site (www.airtran.com).
Alaska Airlines Web site (www.alaskair.com).
America West Airlines Web site (www.americawest.com).
American Medical Women's Association Web site (www.amwa-doc.org)
American Trans Air Web site (www.ata.com).
Amtrak Web site (www.amtrak.com).
Baymont Inns Web site (www.baymontinns.com).
Cheap Tickets Web site (www.cheaptickets.com).
ClubHouse Inns Web site (www.clubhouseinn.com).
Comfort Inns Web site (www.comfortinn.com).
Country Inns and Suites Web site (www.countryinns.com).
Courtyard Marriott Web site (www.courtyard.com).
Days Inns Web site (www.daysinn.com).
Econo Lodge Web site (www.hotelchoice.com).
Encore Web site (www.encoremarketing.com).
Entertainment Publications Web site (www.entertainment.com).
Expedia Web site (www.expedia.com).
Fairfield Inn Web site (www.marriotthotels.com).
Frommer A. "Upstart Airlines Offer Downscale Fares," *Los Angeles Times*, May 14, 2000.
Frontier Airlines Web site (www.frontierairlines.com).
Hampton Inn Web site (www.hampton-inn.com).
Holiday Inn Web site (www.ichotelsgroup.com).
Hostels.com Web site (www.hostels.com).
Hotel Discounts.com Network Web site (www.hoteldiscount.com).
Howard Johnsons Hotels and Inns Web site (www.hojo.com).
JetBlue Airways Web site (www.jetblue.com).
La Quinta Inns Web site (www.laquinta.com).
LowestFare.com Web site (www.lowestfare.com).
Midwest Express Web site (www.midwestexpress.com).
Motel 6 Web site (www.motel6.com).
Orbitz Web site (www.orbitz.com).
Priceline.com Web site (www.priceline.com).
Quikbook Web site (www.quikbook.com).

Ramada Ltd. Web site (www.ramada.com).

Red Roof Inns Web site (www.redroof.com).

Rodeway Inns Web site (www.rodeway.com).

Southwest Airlines Web site (www.iflyswa.com).

Spirit Airlines Web site (www.spiritair.com).

Sun Country Airlines Web site (www.suncountry.com).

Super 8 Web site (www.super8.com).

Teison H, Dunnan N. *Travel Smarts.* Guilford, CT: The Globe Pequot Press, 1999.

Travelocity Web site (www.travelocity.com).

Travelodge Web site (www.travelodge.com).

United Airlines Web site (www.ual.com).

University of California at San Francisco School of Medicine. *The Next Step: Your Guide to Residency.* San Francisco: University of California at San Francisco, 1995.

NOTES

CHAPTER 11

Interview Day

Orient yourself immediately to the interview schedule.

Be prepared by reading up on the program.

The interview process enables you to come to life in the minds of program directors and faculty. So if you have a strong record and good letters of recommendation, you are likely to receive a "halo effect" during the interview process—you will generally be seen in a favorable light. If your record is weaker than you would like, however, the interview may help showcase your personal qualities and commitment to do better.

In the interview, you are given an opportunity to express your commitment to the field to which you are applying and to demonstrate enthusiasm for the program you are visiting. The advice given below applies to all specialties. When you are interviewing for highly competitive positions, however—such as those in dermatology and ophthalmology—questions and processes may become more discriminating as program directors try to distinguish one outstanding student from another.

Review All Program Information

If you are interviewing with several programs over a few days, be sure you don't mix facts about one program with those of another. One very common interview question—"Why have you chosen to apply to this program?"—requires knowledge of the strengths of the program itself. Always prepare an answer for this question in advance. Good answers to this question might be the excellent variety of clinical experiences; the fact that the program is affiliated with a university, VA, community, or county hospital; the breadth of electives offered; the research opportunities available; or the outstanding specialty divisions. You are visiting the program to learn about it and to assess its strengths and weaknesses, but be prepared to demonstrate your favorable impression of the program even early on in the interview day. You can change your mind later, but for now, keep it positive.

Review All Information You Have Submitted

This is a common shortcoming that is frequently observed in student interviews. Be familiar with every detail of what you have said about yourself. Review the file you have prepared. Think of your CV as a menu of topics that your interviewer might choose to discuss. If your CV says that you participated in a research study that was published, be prepared to discuss that research in a polished manner. If you were a member of the internal medicine interest group, be prepared to describe what that group actually did. Bring copies of your CV, personal statement, board scores, and literature about the residency program with you on the interview day. You never know when you might have some downtime, and refreshing your knowledge of the program demonstrates interest and enthusiasm. Also, someone at the program may request to see your application materials during the interview day. Before the big day, you should also get in touch with residents or faculty with ties to your home institution. They may be more open with you about the virtues of the program than people with whom you don't share a common link.

Each program you visit may organize its interview day differently. Much of the tone of the day will also depend on the competitiveness of the situation. For example, many primary care residency programs will use their time to attract you to their programs and make you feel good about yourself and your opportunities. Obviously, a program that matches with just the right number of applicants will not want to risk turning applicants off by asking difficult patient management questions. On the other hand, a competitive program in neurosurgery may design their interview day in a manner that will help sort one applicant from another as efficiently as possible. During all interview activities, applicants must balance making a good impression with finding out everything they can about the program in a short period of time (see Table 11-1). Remember that the evaluation process will continue. Get contact information for helpful residents to use later on in the process. Find out if second, more informal interviews or revisits are welcomed, as these often cement favorable impressions. Usual activities include the following:

- **Preinterview social events.** Some programs may arrange dinner the night before the interview with one or more members of the house staff. These dinners are usually casual but do vary from one program to another. Informal conversation and frank questions about resident satisfaction with the program are appropriate, but bear in mind that you are potentially being evaluated by house staff. This is a time when everyone tends to be positive; more objective evaluation will come later. That being said, use common sense. Stay away from alcohol, mind your table manners, and don't order the most expensive items on the menu. These events may be social (residents only) or more formal extensions of the interview visit (faculty-sponsored). Find out ahead of time and be prepared. Also make an effort to know the dress code. For some affairs, jeans are appropriate; for others, more formal attire may be required.

- **Introduction and orientation.** Larger programs in particular may have interviewees start out together to be addressed by the department chairman or the residency program director. This is a time to get a feel for the overall tone and philosophy of the program. Consider it a plus when the chairman shows an interest in the recruitment effort. The chairman controls the budget, faculty, and resources of a program, and some are more interested in residents than others. The general orientation meeting is usually a time to keep a low profile and listen.

- **Morning rounds and conferences.** Applicants are usually invited to attend morning report or other conferences. Again, this can be an excellent learning experience. Such conferences go on just as they would if guests were not attending. You can therefore judge the value of morning report as

Watch what you say to whom. Assume everyone you meet will have a hand in the rank.

Stay away from alcohol! You need to be in your best form at preinterview social events.

INTERVIEW DAY

TABLE 11-1. Sights to See on a Program Tour

MUST SEE	SHOULD SEE	MIGHT SEE
Wards	Emergency room	Surrounding city
ICU	Cafeteria	Fitness facilities
Surgical suites	Library/computer resources	Child care facilities
Call rooms		

a learning experience, see how faculty and residents interact, and assess the spirit of the house staff in an important activity. On rare occasions, if you are appropriately encouraged and have a valid point to make, you may also participate as you would as a student in your own conferences. As a general rule, however, a low profile is the best approach.

- **Lunch with residents or faculty.** For those who may have missed the preinterview social events, lunch can be a chance to get to know the residents and get a better feel for the program. Use proper table manners and don't eat too much. You don't want to run to the restroom or suffer a post-meal crash in the middle of afternoon activities.

INTERVIEWING

In almost all studies on resident selection, the interview is judged to be one of the most important factors influencing house staff selection. Indeed, specific studies from most disciplines rank the interview at the top of the list or second only to grade point average. Applicant characteristics felt to be important in the interview include compatibility with the program, the ability to articulate thoughts and goals, the ability to work with a team, maturity, and hard work. It should also be noted that medical students find the interview process to be an extremely important element figuring in their selection decisions. "Perceived happiness of current resident" is one of the most important considerations for students, and this assessment is generally made on interview day.

Try to arrive 10 to 15 minutes early on the day of the interview. If possible, make a trial run to the interview location the night before so that you don't get lost or delayed the next day. Punctuality is critical as a resident, and you don't want to make a bad impression to start off your interview day.

Students should also recognize that programs seldom attempt to standardize interviewing techniques from one faculty member to another or even to ask similar questions. Instead, interviews are usually quite informal. However, most will result in some type of quantitative rating that will be included in an overall point score.

Before an actual interview begins, learn the pronunciation of your interviewer's name from the departmental secretary or the interviewer's administrative assistant. Turn down offers for coffee or other drinks; you will be better off not having to worry about what to do with your coffee cup as you are led into your interview. It may help allay anxiety to remember that interviews often run behind schedule and that experienced interviewers are aware of this tendency. If you are running late, your subsequent interviewer will understand when you explain that your previous interview has just concluded. When you meet your interviewer, introduce yourself and offer a firm, confident handshake. Remember to smile and conduct yourself with confidence and poise. After you are invited into the office, do not sit down until the interviewer takes a seat or invites you to do so.

During the interview, maintain fairly constant eye contact with the interviewer. Do not let your gaze or attention wander, especially when the interviewer is speaking directly to you. Do **not** take notes during the interview; instead, remember to write them down later. Try to project a high energy level even if this is your fifteenth interview. Lack of enthusiasm is the most common mistake students make. Many students complain that the most difficult

Table Manners 101.
Always place your napkin in your lap, don't talk with your mouth full, and use utensils, not your fingers.

Apathy is the kiss of death at interview time.

218

interviews are those with faculty members who lack enthusiasm. In fact, this will be the student's greatest challenge. Answer questions fully, but do not ramble; if the interviewer wants to know more about a particular subject, he or she will ask. Speak clearly and use proper grammar. If you can, command the interview toward your strong points, but do not pressure the interviewer or dominate the dialogue. **Never** look at your watch even if you know that the interview is running overtime. When the interview is finished, thank the interviewer, shake hands again, and leave gracefully.

THE INTERVIEW: WHAT CAN BE GAINED

It may be useful to think of the interview as offering specific potential benefits to applicants. These benefits include:

- An opportunity to express enthusiasm for the specialty to which you have committed.
- An opportunity to express enthusiasm for the specific program to which you are applying and to gain a deeper understanding of the strengths of that program.
- A chance to express important character traits that are valued by programs, particularly hard work, endurance, and teamwork.
- A way to provide evidence that one has been well trained with good faculty mentors and role models—i.e., that one comes from a medical school that has provided an environment of excellence.

Depending on the questions asked, most students will have the opportunity to make these points and reap these rewards.

The following are generally **not** useful in the interview process:

- An explanation of why class rank, grade point average, or USMLE scores were not higher.
- A description of any deficiencies in one's medical school as an explanation for a deficiency that a candidate might have.

POPULAR INTERVIEW QUESTIONS AND THE RIGHT ANSWERS!

Although you may be advised about myriad potential interview questions, the following are the only ones that are really common.

1. Why have you chosen this field?

This is the mother of all questions. Programs seek to fill their positions with highly dedicated individuals who are likely to complete their residency training. They do so in the knowledge that if a resident decides he or she does not like surgery, it will be relatively difficult to find a second-year person to fill that resident's slot. Thus, first and foremost to many residency program directors is the student's commitment to and enthusiasm for the specialty. Program directors are very concerned about students who have applied to more than one specialty in the Match.

For these reasons, this is not a time to express indecision even if the choice was difficult. Instead, review your personal statement, as it is likely to hold the answer to this question. Lifestyle and salary are not good reasons for a specialty choice. If this was a factor in your decision, it's better to keep that to

Lifestyle and money are shallow reasons for entering a specialty.

yourself. A radiologist in a small town may take calls every night, and an internist may work in a clinic from eight to five. Few emergency room physicians feel they have chosen a career with an easy lifestyle, although many students may have been told otherwise.

Although the right answers to this question lie largely with the individual, they are likely to include enthusiasm for a particular type of science or service as well as positive experiences in clerkships or electives. Long-standing interest in a field is reassuring as well, as would be the case for a physics major who chooses radiation oncology, a psychology major choosing psychiatry, or a family physician with a long-term commitment to rural areas.

2. Why are you applying to this program?

Stress philosophies and goals also shared by the program.

Although this question is simple and obvious (much like "Why do you want this job?"), many students find themselves unprepared for it. There is, of course, an explanation. Students may be applying to 25 programs, or perhaps they are just beginning the interview process. A program may even have been chosen primarily for geographic reasons or as a fallback. However, this is obviously not what a program director wants to hear. Instead, you must be prepared to enthusiastically describe why the program for which you are interviewing fills your needs. Toward this end, you should be able to find shared philosophies and goals. To do so, however, you must first be familiar with the strengths of the program. It is certainly acceptable to state that "I like this city," "I was born here," or "I have family here," but such responses are not enough; something more specific about the program itself must be included in your response.

3. What are your strengths and weaknesses?

Always choose a weakness that you can spin.

Strengths are easy to describe; after all, you are an elite scholar who was admitted to medical school and is close to graduation. Friends—particularly those outside the profession—would see you as highly disciplined, self-sacrificing, wise, and extremely dedicated. So be prepared to articulate the ways in which you have grown to take pride in yourself and in your work.

Addressing your weaknesses is somewhat trickier. Do not give up too much here: If you tire easily, are readily bored, are unable to function without sleep, or are overly anxious, keep it to yourself, as there is nothing to be gained by confessing your concerns about how you will respond to the difficult year ahead. At the same time, it is hard to state that you are unaware that you possess any weaknesses at all. Common answers are just fine: I am sometimes too intense; I spend too much time in the hospital; I take everything too seriously; I am a perfectionist. You get the idea!

4. Tell me about yourself/tell me about your career plans.

Given that this is often the first question posed in the interview, students should be prepared to discuss both their career goals and other interests. The more specific the plans, the better—e.g., I want to do a cardiology fellowship after my residency and spend part of my time teaching residents and fellows. If your long-term plans are not yet well established, however, it is probably better to state as much.

5. What are you looking for in a residency program?

As with the question "Why did you choose to apply to this program," residency program directors pose the question above because they want to find students who will be happy in their program. Good morale is key to a successful residency program. Thus, excessive concern about salary or work hours will not be seen as positive. You will earn respect by seeking to ensure that the board pass rate is high, that education is a priority, that all ACGME (Accreditation Council for Graduate Medical Education) requirements for that specialty are being met, and that residents are of high quality. If you are going into a primary care field, you will also want a program that has a great continuity clinic. If you are entering a surgery field, you should be concerned about case mix.

In addition to the above questions, there are interview questions common to each specialty. See Table 11-2.

TABLE 11-2. Commonly Asked Interview Questions by Specialty

SPECIALTY	COMMONLY ASKED QUESTIONS
All specialties	Why did you apply to this program? What are you looking for in a residency program? Why are you interested in this specialty? Where do you see yourself in the future?
Anesthesiology	Why do you want to enter anesthesiology? Why did you apply to our residency program? What do you envision yourself doing after you finish your residency? What other residency programs are you applying to, and why did you choose to apply to these programs?
Dermatology	Have you had any prior research experience in this field? What is your potential contribution to the field?
Diagnostic radiology	Why do you want to enter radiology? Why did you apply to our residency program? What do you envision yourself doing after you finish your residency? What other residency programs are you applying to, and why did you choose to apply to these programs?
Emergency medicine	Why have you chosen a four-year program versus a three-year program (and vice versa)? Why are you interested in emergency medicine? Tell me about an interesting case that you have seen. What are some of your personal strengths and weaknesses? What would you do for a living if you couldn't go into emergency medicine?
Family practice	What is your focus in family practice? How do you feel about specific ethical issues in health care, such as end-of-life issues? Do you feel comfortable working with patients of all ages?

TABLE 11-2. Commonly Asked Interview Questions by Specialty *(continued)*

SPECIALTY	COMMONLY ASKED QUESTIONS
General surgery	Do you enjoy working under pressure?
	Have you done any research in general surgery?
	Tell us about an interesting clinical case that you saw during your general surgery rotation.
	What is your long-term plan?
Internal medicine	What are your personal strengths and weaknesses?
	We're going to give you a clinical scenario and you'll provide the diagnosis.
Medicine-pediatrics	Why med-peds?
	What are your strengths?
	Where do you see your career taking you?
Neurology	What research projects are you involved in?
	Could we have your opinion on an ethical issue?
Neurosurgery	Why neurosurgery?
	What research projects are you involved in?
	Ethics questions may also be asked.
	What is your long-term plan?
OB/GYN	What was the most interesting case that you saw as a medical student during your OB/GYN rotation?
	Have you done any research in OB/GYN? If so, tell me about your research project.
Ophthalmology	Will you answer some clinical questions?
	Do you have any contingency plans?
	What is your research/clinical background?
Orthopedic surgery	Why do you want to enter orthopedics?
	Why did you apply to our residency program?
	What do you envision yourself doing after you finish your residency?
	Have you done any research in orthopedics? If so, tell me about your research project.
Otolaryngology	Why did you choose otolaryngology?
	What are your academic and research interests?
	Tell me about an interesting case.
	Where do you see this practice heading in the future?
	What is your long-term plan?
Pathology	What are your postresidency plans?
	Why have you chosen this field?
Pediatrics	Do you react well with children and their parents?
	Why did you decide to go into pediatrics?
Physical medicine and rehabilitation	What is your focus in physical medicine?
	Do you feel comfortable working with patients of all ages?
	What are your personal strengths and weaknesses?

INTERVIEW DAY

222

TABLE 11-2. Commonly Asked Interview Questions by Specialty *(continued)*

SPECIALTY	COMMONLY ASKED QUESTIONS
Radiation oncology	Are you comfortable handling issues related to death and dying?
	What are your thoughts about euthanasia?
	(May present a clinical scenario around the ethical issues of euthanasia.)
	What are your personal strengths and weaknesses?
Urology	Have you done any research in urology? What kind? Explain.
	Tell us about an interesting clinical case that you saw during your urology rotation.
	What are your personal strengths and weaknesses?

* In all specialties, questions about ethics and legal issues may be asked.

OTHER POTENTIAL INTERVIEW TOPICS

Other topics that sometimes arise are as follows:

1. Describe an interesting case!

It is not common for students to be asked to present or discuss cases, since most faculty members recognize that such questions will make the student uncomfortable and undermine the rapport between student and interviewer. Furthermore, testing medical knowledge on the basis of one case is not productive when grades, USMLE scores, and other data are available. Nevertheless, it is possible that you will be asked to present a case that had a significant bearing on your education, so be sure to have a case memorized! Be ready with a brief presentation and a lesson learned.

Should you have a case presented to you, see if it is intended to test a basic lesson. For example, that lesson might be to not believe every lab test, to ask the patient a question that was missed, to check the physical exam again, or to take the history and do the physical yourself. We do know of some cases that have been presented to students with the goal of testing basic approaches to a patient.

2. Discuss the politics of health care.

Although we have not found this topic to be a significant area for student interviews, it is important to be aware of the challenges health care providers face today. Chairmen and residency program directors will be concerned about how medical education will be funded in the future. They will be concerned about how faculty can generate their own salaries while still finding the time to teach effectively and do research. They will want to provide indigent care but will recognize that academic medical centers cannot care for all patients who lack health insurance. They will seek reform in the medical malpractice process. Be engaging but not overly political in your discussion of these topics.

INTERVIEW DAY

ILLEGAL QUESTIONS

Questions considered illegal in employment screening are those that deal with race, sex, age, body habitus, marital status, family plans, or physical disability. If you are asked an illegal question, don't be defensive. Many faculty may be new to interviewing and may not realize that their question is inappropriate.

In response to an illegal question, you may choose:

1. **To answer.** This is the safest course. You may be open or vague. For example, if asked about plans to start a family, you might answer, "I have no plans to do so until after I complete my training." Another answer could be, "My education is my priority right now."
2. **To deflect.** You can sidestep the question by saying something like, "Interesting question. I haven't really thought about it."
3. **To decline to answer.** You could remind the interviewer that his or her question is illegal and politely refuse to comment. This is a high-risk tactic.

WHAT DO I ASK THE INTERVIEWER?

The questions you ask can be revealing to the interviewer.

Toward the middle or the end of the session, your interviewer will invariably ask you, "Do you have any questions?" Be prepared in advance with at least one or two questions that demonstrate your interest, as long as they are appropriate to the interviewer or to the program. Faculty members can field more philosophical and broad-based questions such as the ones listed below.

An ideal question to ask is one that the interviewer will enjoy answering, thus lending a positive tone to the encounter. Remember, however, that you are still the person under observation and evaluation, so do **not** harp on the program's weaknesses. Also avoid asking questions about salaries and benefits, vacation, moonlighting, call schedules, and other aspects of day-to-day program operations. Save these practical concerns for the house staff, and keep your interview questions friendly and benign. Appropriate questions for faculty interviewers are as follows:

1. Where have your residents gone after graduation?
2. What process do you have for improving the residency? For evaluating rotations? Do you anticipate any changes in the residency program?
3. Have you ever done surveys of your graduates? What do they tell you?
4. What research opportunities are available? What is the availability of funding for research? What kind of mentor support is available from the faculty?
5. In what direction do you see the chairman (or residency director) taking the program? Do you believe that he or she will remain here during my residency training?
6. What opportunities are available to attend regional and national conferences and seminars?
7. How well do residents perform on board certification exams?
8. What is the structure of the last years of residency? Does the program offer elective time? Mini-fellowships? Time and opportunity to work abroad?
9. Is there training relating to the business and legal aspects of the specialty?

We have compiled a list of questions that you might ask house staff while you are visiting the program. Most of these questions deal with the daily operation of the residency. A few questions, however, are sensitive ones that you might not feel comfortable asking all house staff members you encounter (e.g., chief residents steeped in the program's "party line"). Given that any question you ask could potentially make it back to the selection committee, always exercise discretion, especially with touchy topics.

General Questions

1. Are the residents happy? What features of the program do they like or dislike?
2. Would the residents choose the same program again?
3. Does the program have trouble filling all its spots?
4. How strong are the residents? From which institutions did they graduate?

Location

1. Is the program located in a safe part of the city? If not, what is the security system like?
2. What do residents do for fun around here?
3. What advantages are specific to the location (e.g., unusual patient population, cultural opportunities, climate, low cost of living)?

Reputation

1. Do graduates of the program have problems finding jobs?
2. How difficult is it for residents to get a good fellowship?

Education

1. Is the program fully accredited? For how long?
2. How are the residents evaluated? By whom?
3. Is there an organized curriculum? What is its emphasis?
4. How many conferences are there per week? Do conferences emphasize practical knowledge or state-of-the-art research?
5. What is the quality of the attendings? What are their responsibilities? Do they get along?
6. How interested are the faculty in the education and welfare of the house staff?
7. What proportion of attendings are private?
8. Are there medical students on the wards? What school(s) do they represent? What are the residents' teaching responsibilities to the students?
9. What research opportunities are there? Are faculty research preceptors readily available?

Work Environment

1. What is the patient load like?
2. What are the typical admissions diagnoses?

3. How many cases are treated by the average resident?
4. Is the caseload sufficiently varied?
5. How much autonomy do residents have to manage patients?
6. What is the patient population like? Ethnicity/language? Socioeconomic status?
7. Is there continuity of care for patients after discharge?
8. What is the extent and quality of the ambulatory experience?
9. How strong is nursing support? Consult services? Radiology? Pathology? Emergency services?
10. How much "scut work" is done by house staff? Are there blood-drawing/IV teams?
11. What is the typical call schedule?
12. How does the work environment vary from service to service? From hospital to hospital?
13. How busy are call nights? How much sleep do you usually get?
14. How available are the attendings? Can you call them at night?
15. Is there backup available when you're on call? Is there a night float system?
16. How many hours do you work each week?
17. How much time do you get off each week?

Salary

1. What is the starting salary for an intern? For an R2?
2. What about cost of living in the area?
3. Is moonlighting permitted? If so, how does it work around here?

Benefits

1. What health benefits are available (e.g., medical insurance, dental plan, vision plan)? Are spouses covered?
2. What is the maternity/paternity leave policy?
3. Is life insurance available? Disability insurance?
4. Is parking provided? Is subsidized housing available? What is the vacation schedule setup?

If you have a chance, you may also want to speak with senior medical students at the institution you are visiting. They can provide additional insight and perspective into the institution and area.

QUESTIONS FOR THE CHAIRMAN AND PROGRAM DIRECTOR

Department chairmen see the residency program as lying somewhere in a list of priorities. They are also responsible for the overall budget, and their generosity may make the difference between going to a conference or staying home; whether or not an away elective is possible on the basis of funding issues; or whether startup funds are available for a resident research project. Similarly, chairmen will know what changes may be imminent in a program or whether a program is likely to grow or get smaller. They will also be responsible for helping recruit the best possible teaching faculty. Questions about these objectives—e.g., whether additional faculty are being recruited or whether residents are encouraged to do research—will give chairmen an opportunity to discuss their role in the residency program.

The residency program director is the most important person with whom you will interview. It is therefore key to determine if he or she appears to have a genuine concern for residents. If the program director does not demonstrate the personal qualities to treat you well on the interview, the situation will be worse when you arrive for work. Ask about his or her plans for the future, ideas about curricular change, assessment of the quality of the graduating residents, and approach to board preparation.

PROBLEMS WITH THE INTERVIEW

Given all the time, expense, and adrenaline that enter into your program interviews, you don't want to hurt your chances for success with an ill-considered answer or comment. Some of the problems that students face during the interview day are as follows:

- **Underestimating the importance of first impressions.** Before you ever open your mouth to answer a question, you are sending a message to your interviewer. Proper grooming, confident posture, a smile, and a firm handshake are key. You may be nervous, but this is not the time to let it show.

- **Blurting out responses.** If you are blindsided by a difficult question, it's okay to pause for a moment and think before you answer. It may feel long, but taking a few moments to collect yourself can pay off with a smooth answer.

- **Rambling.** Interviewers probably hear enough poorly constructed medical student presentations as it is, so try to focus your responses. If rambling is just a nervous habit for you, the problem should dissipate as you gain experience and become more comfortable with the interview process. If this is not the case, however, you should make a conscious effort to provide complete yet focused answers. You may find that practice sessions with a friendly classmate can help you overcome this tendency.

- **Not knowing anything about the program.** No one will ever expect you to know their programs through and through, but you should at least know the basics of each. Interviewers do not want to waste the time allotted for the interview going over information that is already available in their printed materials.

- **Focusing on the program's weaknesses.** It's true in a philosophical sense that you are interviewing the program as much as they are interviewing you. But be practical; don't put the interviewer on the defensive by concentrating on the program's weaknesses. If these problem spots are of paramount importance to you, save your concerns for the house staff or raise the issue in a friendly, nonconfrontational manner.

- **Inconsistent/evasive answers.** Answers that don't match up with what you wrote on your application will place interviewers on the alert, as will answers that are incomplete. Do emphasize your strengths as well as the clinical and academic interests you share with the interviewer. At the same time, do not exaggerate, lie, or otherwise distort facts. Interviewers expect applicants to be open and honest.

- **Displaying an eccentric personality.** The interviewer is trying to picture you as a junior colleague with whom daily interaction will be necessary. So if you come across as domineering, inflexible, or temperamental, you will hurt your chances of selection even if your grades and other scores are good.

- **Pejorative comments about other programs.** Negative statements (especially unsolicited or unsupported digs) about other programs or your own school will be noted as indiscretions and will reflect badly on you. Inter-

You have put a lot of work into interviewing. Don't cut yourself short by being unprepared.

Don't get lured into criticizing other programs.

viewers will wonder what you might say about their program at the next stop on your tour. You should also remember that the academic community is tight, and the interviewer may have colleagues and friends at the programs you just put down.

- **Poor interactions with administrative or house staff.** It goes without saying that rudeness or lack of consideration for administrative personnel will be relayed to the residency selection committee and will end up as a strike against you. The secretary to the chairman or program director may well relay a respected opinion about you to the boss. Always be on your best behavior and remember your manners in all of your interactions throughout the interview day. It's important to be polite to everyone, not just your interviewers.

- **Not rehearsing answers.** As discussed earlier in this chapter, several interview questions are quite common, and you should have practiced the right answers before the big day. Avoid fumbling by participating in a mock interview session (speak with your adviser). Vary the structure of your answers a little so that you don't come across as rehearsed.

- **Not promoting key assets.** Before you begin interviewing, you should prepare a list of key points that you would like to get across during the course of your interview. You may not have complete control over what is asked of you during the interview, but by knowing beforehand what information you would like to convey, you can work it into your answers.

- **Zoning out.** Now is the time to focus and show that you have good listening skills. If you have adequately prepared for your interview, you won't need to think of how you are going to answer a question while the interviewer is still speaking. Avoid the embarrassment of not addressing a question properly by concentrating on what your interviewer is saying.

- **Selling yourself short.** You should avoid rambling, but never give a "yes" or "no" answer to an interviewer's questions. Always follow up with something that emphasizes your strengths as an applicant.

- **Sticking your foot in your mouth.** A little silence is okay during the interview. If you finish answering a question and are met with a blank stare, don't panic. The interviewer may be taking a mental note or thinking of what to ask you next, or he or she may be trying to make you nervous. Avoid the temptation to change your answer or say something stupid.

- **Minding your manners—to the extreme.** It is important to be polite and formal, but not to the point that you avoid making a connection with your interviewer. Don't be so focused on professionalism that you come across as rigid and distant. Relax a little and enjoy getting to know your interviewer.

- **Being apathetic.** People who volunteer to interview do so because they are excited about their program and their specialty. They are looking for applicants who share the same enthusiasm. If you are jet-lagged, feeling blue, or having a slow morning, put that aside and focus on being the animated, energetic person that they might want to work with some day.

- **Lacking confidence.** If you have made it to the interview, you are past the hurdle of being considered acceptable. Don't let the stress of the interview day or the competition get the best of you. Remind yourself of how far you have come, and go on your selling points. Projecting poise requires more than speaking confidently. Remember nonverbal cues as well: be certain to stand tall, smile, offer a firm handshake, don't fiddle or fidget, and maintain eye contact.

- **Lacking interest.** Even if all your questions have been answered a hundred times over, never say no when an interviewer asks if you have any questions. It is always of benefit to get different perspectives on aspects of the program, and not asking a question could lead the interviewer to think that you are not very interested in the program.

- **Ending on a low note.** The end to the interview should mirror the beginning. Eye contact, a smile, and a firm handshake, together with thanking the interviewer for his or her time, are critical for a memorable finish.

WRAPPING UP THE INTERVIEW DAY

If you are serious about a program and want to learn more about it, speak to the departmental secretary or a house staff member about possible arrangements for a return visit. This will allow you to spend more time on rounds, in clinic or surgery, in conferences, and in the surrounding neighborhood. It will also give you an opportunity to confirm or modify your initial impressions of the program. A second visit can be extremely helpful to you and will also confirm to the program that you are interested in it. Practically, you will probably be able to do only one or two return visits, so save such visits for the programs in which you are most interested.

Be sure to jot down your impressions of each program while they are still fresh in your mind. After you have visited four or five programs, the details will start to blur. To help keep your facts and impressions straight, write down all your thoughts about a program as soon as you can at the end of the day. Use the Program Evaluation Worksheet provided in Appendix C if you need something to organize your thoughts. You will thank yourself later when you can rank your programs with organized notes while your classmates are banging their heads against the wall trying to remember which program had the deluxe call rooms with the well-stocked refrigerators and HBO.

Also make a point of evaluating your own performance during the interview. If you were surprised by a question, review how you might give a more polished answer. If you had any difficulties, review the *Problems with the Interview* section and take steps to ensure a better interview at the next program.

FOLLOW-UP LETTERS

Unless your interviewer explicitly tells you not to do so, write a letter to thank the program for its hospitality as well as to express your continued interest. This typed letter should be composed and mailed no more than a few days after the interview, while memories of the interview (on your part and theirs) are still fresh. A sincere follow-up letter can help solidify the impression you left on the interviewer before it is washed away by subsequent interviews.

Personalize your letter by mentioning a specific topic that was discussed during the interview. If you recently received any honors or awards, you can use your letter to update your application file. The letter should be addressed to your interviewers. Do not be shy in describing why you liked the program and in stating that you will be ranking it highly—if in fact you plan to do so (see Figure 11-1). It should be noted, however, that follow-up letters carry limited weight, as many applicants choose to follow up on all the programs in which they interviewed. Program directors are thus skeptical of follow-up letters in general.

Have follow-up letters in the mail within 1–2 days of the interview.

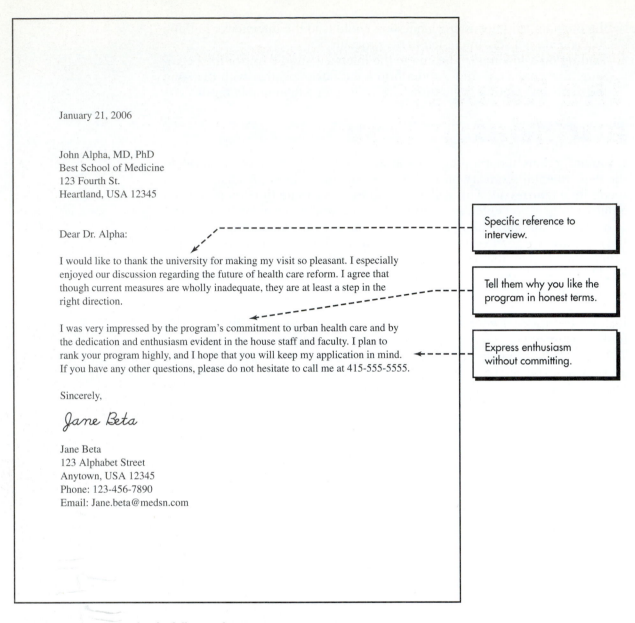

January 21, 2006

John Alpha, MD, PhD
Best School of Medicine
123 Fourth St.
Heartland, USA 12345

Dear Dr. Alpha:

I would like to thank the university for making my visit so pleasant. I especially
enjoyed our discussion regarding the future of health care reform. I agree that
though current measures are wholly inadequate, they are at least a step in the
right direction.

I was very impressed by the program's commitment to urban health care and by
the dedication and enthusiasm evident in the house staff and faculty. I plan to
rank your program highly, and I hope that you will keep my application in mind.
If you have any other questions, please do not hesitate to call me at 415-555-5555.

Sincerely,

Jane Beta

Jane Beta
123 Alphabet Street
Anytown, USA 12345
Phone: 123-456-7890
Email: Jane.beta@medsn.com

Specific reference to interview.

Tell them why you like the program in honest terms.

Express enthusiasm without committing.

FIGURE 11-1. Example of a follow-up letter.

References

Crane JT, Ferraro CM. Selection criteria for emergency medicine residency applicants. *Acad Emerg Med* 7(1):54–60, 2000.

Delisa JA, Jain SS, Campagnolo DI. Factors used by physical medicine and rehabilitation residency training directors to select their residents. *Am J Phys Med Rehabil* 73(3):152–156, 1994.

Pretorius ES, Hrung J. Factors that affect National Resident Matching Program rankings of medical students applying for radiology residency. *Acad Radiol* 9(1):75–81, 2002.

Taylor CA, Weinstein L, Mayhew HE. The process of resident selection: a view from the residency director's desk. *Obstet Gynecol* 85(2):299–303, 1995.

Wagoner NE, Suriano JR. Program directors' responses to a survey on variables used to select residents in a time of change. *Acad Med* 74(1):51–58, 1999.

Wagoner NE, Suriano JR, Stoner JA. Factors used by program directors to select residents. *J Med Educ* 61(1):10–21, 1986.

The Rank List and Match Day

Do not rush the rank. It is a decision you'll have to live with for a long time.

Even before the dust settles from the whirlwind of interview season, you will be faced with a still more challenging task: creating your rank-order list (ROL). Year after year, really smart applicants make regrettable mistakes when it comes to ranking programs. These missteps can only shortchange the applicant. To clarify the ranking process, we have developed two rules—and only two—to remember when you create your ROL.

Rule #1: Rank programs in order of their desirability. Desirability combines what you, the applicant, consider to be your true preference for residency with the strength of an individual program as it relates to your residency training. Since you have already deeply scrutinized all the programs across the country while determining where to apply and subsequently interview, the process now focuses on your interpretation of the desirability of each program. Look back through all the notes you took along the interview trail, remembering your gut feeling at each place and your interactions with residents and faculty. Some might find it helpful to make a list of pros and cons when faced with close ranking decisions, while others might need only a few minutes of reflection to solidify the "best" order. Remember, your ROL need not mirror the "Top 10" from any source other than your own head. The object is to match with your most desirable program, not to match with your first-ranked choice.

Ideally, the programs at the bottom of your ROL will serve as backups—acceptable programs that are a sure bet. Do not rank a program lower because you believe your chances of attaining that program are slim. The ROL is private and transient. You don't have to show yours to anyone, and once the Match is over, it will never be seen again. So this is the time to shoot high—don't sell yourself short, but be prepared for the unexpected as well. This caveat brings us to the second rule.

Rule #2: Rank all acceptable programs. After you have completed your interviews, you should have only two categories of programs: acceptable and unacceptable. **Do not rank any programs in which you would not be willing to work.** Remember that you are under contract to report to the program in which you match. If the program is on your ROL at all, you're telling the National Residency Matching Program (NRMP) that you are willing to go to that program if you match there. You are under no obligation to rank every program that you visit. However, you must decide whether it is better to match at a less-than-ideal program or take your chances in the Scramble if you do not match. The latter option, while highly undesirable, is certainly viable in specialties that often have a large number of unfilled positions on Match Day, such as family medicine or internal medicine.

The actual number of programs to rank depends on several factors, including the competitiveness of the specialty, the competition for the specific programs being ranked, and the applicant's qualifications. In most instances, the issue is not the actual number of programs on the ROL, but whether to add one or more programs to the list in order to reduce the likelihood of being unmatched. Both applicants and programs are well advised to include all acceptable choices on their ROLs. A long ROL in no way affects the chances of being matched to choices higher on the ROL. It is interesting to note, however, that U.S. seniors consistently have the highest Match rate and the longest av-

THE RANK LIST AND MATCH DAY

erage ROLs. Although there are small year-to-year variations, about 95% of U.S. seniors match each year.

For students applying in extremely competitive fields such as orthopedics or dermatology, following these rules too strictly can lead to heartbreak. The intense competition in some specialties means that unless you walk on water, it is possible that you will not get a match. To prepare for such a competitive match, students should carefully consider the value of applying to positions outside their specialty of choice. If not matching is unacceptable, it would be wise to have a backup plan in another field, whether this includes scrambling for a different residency specialty or applying for a year of post-doctoral research.

The two rules above do not guarantee a match; they guarantee only that you will do the best you can with the tools you have at your disposal. If you are having a tough time putting all your information together, walk through your ROL with your significant other, friend, or career adviser. See Table 12-1 for a summary of ways to improve your chances of matching.

The NRMP Matching Algorithm

The algorithm used by the NRMP is the same as that used by the Canadian Resident Matching Service. Outlined below is a simplified explanation of the NRMP algorithm. For details (or to view a sample match between five students and five programs), visit the NRMP Web site at www.nrmp.org/res_match/about_res/algorithms.html.

1. The process begins with an attempt to place an applicant into his or her first-choice program. If a match cannot be made because the program is already filled (with more desirable applicants) or the applicant was not ranked by that program, an attempt is then made to match with the next program on his or her ROL. Note that the second program on the ROL is now treated as that applicant's *first* choice in the Match. This process continues until a tentative match has been made or the applicant is left unmatched.
2. In the next round, an attempt is made to place the next applicant into his or her first-choice program. If this new applicant is more attractive to a program than another applicant who is already tentatively matched, the least preferred applicant is removed to make room for the more desirable applicant, and a new tentative match is made. The process will be repeated for the candidate who was removed from the Match.
3. The process is carried out for all applicants until each has been tentatively matched to the most preferred choice possible or until all choices have been exhausted.

TABLE 12-1. Ways to Improve Your Chances of Matching

Realistically assess your competitiveness and the competitiveness of the programs.
Apply and interview at a sufficient number of programs.
Rank all programs acceptable to you.
If you aim for a tough specialty, have a backup.

4. When all applicants have been considered, the tentative matches become final and the process is complete.

In short, each applicant moves "down" his or her ROL until a tentative match has been made or all choices have been exhausted, while each program moves "up" its ROL. Note that no applicant can be bypassed by a lower-ranked applicant for a given program. If the higher-ranked applicant did not match there, it's because the applicant already had a more desirable offer in hand. Since the algorithm was computerized in 1974, the process takes only minutes to run each year—but we still wait weeks to find out the results!

How Do Couples Rank Programs?

The NRMP Handbook for Students includes a step-by-step guide for creating a couples ROL that is quite extensive and is generally sound. In general, the goal of the couples Match is for you and your partner to stay geographically close to one another. This is a good time to reiterate that any two people can register in the couples Match. Marriage, sexual orientation, medical school attended, and field of interest are not considered by the computer algorithm in the couples Match.

That said, you and your partner should first-rank programs as if you were matching on your own. Turn to "How Do I Rank the Programs?" for guidelines (see above). You should then list the possible program pairs if you are ranking more than one program in the same city. In addition to program pairs in the same city/area (Type 1), there are two other types of program pairs to consider: pairs of programs not in the same city/area (Type 2) and combinations in which one partner goes unmatched (Type 3). Consider creating and ranking Type 2 pairings if separation is tolerable. These pairs allow both partners to match semi-independently. Because Type 2 pairings are not restricted by geography, the number of possible permutations is large. Consider creating and ranking Type 3 pairings if it is acceptable for one of you to match and the other to enter the Scramble. This is usually preferable to both of you going unmatched.

Ranking programs as a couple is an exercise in communication and compromise.

Ranking program pairs is a classic process of give-and-take. Fortunately, the process can be less painful if you and your partner have communicated well during the application process and thus have an understanding of one another's preferences. Couples must decide how much weight to give to location as opposed to programs. Regardless, the process may take a few evenings. After all, your ROL can easily be more than 100 pairs long. When ranking Type 3 pairings, you should also factor in the location, as it will be easier for the unmatched partner to scramble in a large city with many training programs. You can register for the couples Match when both of you enter your ROLs. You must have your partner's Association of American Medical Colleges (AAMC) ID number, and he or she will appear as a "linked" Match list.

As with the regular Match, you should keep in mind that it is possible that you, your partner, or both may not match at any of your ranked programs. You should discuss this possibility and think through the different scenarios if the worst comes to pass. Coordination, communication, and a good action plan are critical for a couple in the Scramble (see below).

Supplemental Rank-Order Lists

When an applicant ranks an advanced position (which begins 15 months after the Match), he or she also submits a ranking of PGY-1 (transitional or preliminary) programs on a supplemental rank-order list (SROL). The applicant can submit more than one SROL, thus tailoring PGY-1 preferences to the location of the advanced training. If you do not match into an advanced position, your SROLs will not be used. If you go unmatched on your SROL, your advanced Match result still holds. You can rank up to 15 programs on your SROLs combined at no charge.

"We Are Ranking You at the Top of Our List" (Not!)

Programs often send candidates follow-up letters after an interview to confirm or feel out their interest in the program. While applicants and program directors may express a high degree of interest in each other and try to influence a decision in their favor, they must not make statements implying a commitment. Follow-up letters often contain statements that can be misinterpreted by either party. Sometimes program directors may even assure you that you will be ranked at the top of their list. While such information may be flattering, do **not** count on it, and do **not** let it affect your ROL. If a program says that you will be ranked first, all it means is that you can match no lower than that program. Some applicants have an instinctive but unfortunate tendency to favor programs that they believe are more likely to accept them. Others allow these follow-up letters to limit the length of their ROL inappropriately. Again, **all** acceptable programs should be on your ROL.

Under-the-Table Deals

In some of the more competitive fields, program directors or department chairmen may call applicants after the interview but before Match Day to ask about their ranking of the program. **It is a violation of Match rules for programs to ask you (or vice versa) for this information.** (Applicants might consider reporting the incident to your dean of students, the NRMP, or the appropriate specialty board after the Match.) That being said, the Match Participation Agreement does not prohibit either party from making such statements, but such declarations do have consequences. Thus, unless the caller represents your top choice, this question is only a golden opportunity for you to hang yourself. If you tell the program you are not ranking them first, they might drop you on their ROL to ensure that they get their top picks. Believe it or not, some programs would rather minimize how low they go on their ROL than just go for their top candidates. If the caller is from one of your top choices, **get a commitment in writing from the residency director.** If he or she balks, then all bets are off. All in all, it is best to simply tell the soliciting program that you expect to rank them very highly, even if you do not intend to do so. Beware that telling multiple programs you will rank them first may come back to haunt you; program directors often talk to each other, and your credibility rating will soon be in the dumpster if word gets out that you have told more than one location they are your "number one pick." It is important to remember that the faculty who help choose the ROL for the program you match with will ultimately be your colleagues, and breaking trust among work partners across the country is a poor way to start any business.

Enter "out of Match" deals with caution.

It has been noted that several programs—especially those in fields that traditionally do not fill, such as pathology and family medicine—are increasingly using "under-the-table" negotiating to recruit international medical graduates (IMGs). They see these applicants as less choosy than U.S. medical graduates and therefore think they can "lock in" a good applicant from abroad by offering him or her a deal outside the Match. If you find yourself in this situation, carefully consider what is to be gained and lost from such an agreement. On the one hand, it is nice to have a guaranteed position in the United States. On the other hand, if you are being offered a position outside the Match, it is likely that other programs will find you equally desirable, so you might fare well at a higher choice if you went through the Match. In the end, the final decision is yours—but without a contract and at least some discussion of visa and licensure issues (see Chapter 5), you should not even consider withdrawing from the main Match.

Entering Your ROL

As of the 1999 Match, all ROLs for specialties participating in the NRMP Match must be submitted electronically through the Internet using the Rank-Order List and Input Confirmation (ROLIC) system. You will indicate your preferences from among the programs at which you interviewed, which are each identified by a specific program code. Programs entered into the ROLIC system may include preliminary or transitional, categorical, or advanced programs or a combination of these. Make sure you double check that the code you listed on the ROLIC system completely matches your desired program. You can also list several different specialty types (e.g., internal medicine, family practice, surgery). If you rank advanced (PGY-2) positions on your ROL and wish to secure a first-year (PGY-1) position as well, you will also be required to submit an SROL. Note that you will be charged additional fees for ranking more than 15 programs. More detailed information can be found in the NRMP Handbook for Students or on the NRMP Web site (www.nrmp. org).

Students applying to specialties that have their own Match must send their ROL to their specific matching program. Contact information for these specialties is provided in Chapter 1.

Finalizing or turning in your ROL can feel like asking someone to marry you. You're absolutely sure until the moment you turn in that piece of paper. Then you start thinking, "Wait a minute . . . did I do the right thing?" Most of the soul searching and turmoil you experience will focus on the ordering of your top three choices. Discuss the strengths and weaknesses of these three programs with your significant other or close friend.

Only certified lists are used in the Match. When applicants have finished entering their lists, they must certify them by clicking on a button and entering their NRMP password to confirm it. Changes can be made to the ROL after it has been certified. This gives applicants a way to "try out" a ranking order for a few days while retaining the option of changing it in the future—as long as the deadline has not passed. **However, once the list has been changed, the new version must be certified in order to be used in the Match.** Changes include adding a program to the list, deleting a program from the list, and changing the order of the programs. Please note that the system does not retain previous versions of the rank list, so the list displayed on the screen upon logging in is the only version on file with the NRMP.

Is it too late to modify the ROL after you have turned it in and the deadline is passed? Actually, it is not too late. The NRMP will accept faxed changes for a few days after the deadline has passed if your dean of students makes a request on your behalf. But this option is disruptive and depends heavily on your dean, so don't view it as an opportunity to mull over your ROL past the deadline. Use this option only as a last resort—and only with good reason.

Getting Out of the Match

While all applicants and programs who enter into the Match agree to a binding commitment, there are extenuating circumstances of serious hardship wherein a waiver may be granted.

"Serious hardship" refers to the occurrence of a highly unusual, unexpected, and unpredictable situation or circumstance that renders the fulfillment of the Match obligation impossible or would result in irreparable harm to any one of the committed Match participants.

Examples of serious hardship include an applicant who failed to graduate on time; the closing of a program or institution; the death or serious illness of a family member that requires the applicant to alter the choice of residency location; or the loss of accreditation by a program or institution. It does **not** include taking advantage of a more desirable program or applicant after the ROLs are submitted.

MARCH MATCHNESS ("IT'S AWESOME, BABY!")

The NRMP Match itself is run in late February. The results are known to your dean's office several days before Match Day, which is usually on a Thursday in mid-March. The Monday before Match Day at 12 noon is the moment of truth for most. If you do not hear from your dean's office during this period, you can assume that you matched. You can also log in to the NRMP's Registration, Ranking, and Results (R3) System using your AAMC ID and password. One of six messages will have been sent to your account, stating that you have either matched (fully, to an advanced but not a first-year position, to a first-year position only) or not matched (in any category, due either to a noncertified list or to being withdrawn). If you did match, then you must wait until Match Day itself to find out where you matched. If you do learn that you have not matched, read on for information about the Scramble.

Prank calls pretending to be the dean's office on Unmatch Day are not funny.

A list of matched independent applicants by code is published on Unmatch Day (the day before Match Day). If you are an independent candidate and your code is **not** listed, call the NRMP after 9 a.m. Eastern Standard Time (EST) to confirm your Match status.

At medical schools on Match Day, the results are announced simultaneously across the nation at noon EST. Many schools organize ceremonies or more casual breakfasts around this event; applicants often bring their significant others to provide moral support and to share in the anticipation. The atmosphere is usually electric by the time the signal is given to open the envelope.

If this is a moment that you would rather not share with your entire medical school class, the results of the Match are usually available online an hour later, around 1 p.m. EST.

If the news is bad, the fact that you did not match does not amount to a personal rejection from the entire medical profession. It might help your bruised ego to recognize that failure to match most often results from a poorly thought-out ROL or simply from applying either to a small number of programs or to programs within a highly competitive specialty. It might also be comforting to know that you are not alone; approximately 1000 U.S. medical students and several thousand non-U.S. medical student applicants enter the Scramble each year, and most find quality residency positions immediately.

Now is not the time to panic.
Relax and focus.
The Scramble begins at noon
EST on Unmatch Day.

You will have to postpone your moping and self-pity until later. Things will begin to happen very quickly during the "Scramble" period, which lasts from 12 noon EST (no earlier!) on the third Tuesday in March, until 12 noon on the third Thursday in March each year. First, you will be apprised of your situation by your dean either on Unmatch Day or the day before, or you may find out from your account on the NRMP site. At this time, the NRMP also releases the Dynamic List of Unfilled Positions, accessible through the NRMP Web site and updated every hour to reflect the number of remaining unfilled positions. You may be able to meet with your adviser or your department chairman who can contact program directors on your behalf. ERAS is also available to those who have participated in ERAS during the regular season and who have paid their account in full no less than two weeks prior to the Scramble period. These applicants can use ERAS to apply to a maximum of 30 programs free of charge.

If your adviser is unavailable or if you are not a U.S. medical student, you may have to contact the programs directly. After you make your list of programs in order of interest, track down the program phone numbers in AMA-FREIDA or the "Green Book." You can also look up the area code of that program and call information, (area code) 555-1212, to get a local number, or you can refer to the program's Web site. You will then need to assemble the following documents for a faxable application file (especially if you are not using the ERAS system):

- Dean's letter
- Transcript
- A copy of the NRMP Universal Application/ERAS application
- Your CV (ERAS provides a printable CV)
- Any letters of recommendation that you may have

You are not restricted to programs in a previously selected specialty. Many applicants decide to pursue additional programs in another specialty because there are too few Scramble positions available in their initial specialty selection (e.g., surgery).

Begin your quest by calling programs in the order in which they appear on your hot list starting at noon EST on Unmatch Day (the day before Match Day). The day will be hectic and stressful, so steel yourself for busy signals and harried program secretaries, and make a conscious effort to remain calm and friendly. You will need to fax your application file to interested programs. Your dean's office or the department in your specialty should give you full access to their phones and fax machines. Positions will be offered by phone. If you are offered a position at a program that is low on your hot list, ask them how long they are willing to hold that position for you. Otherwise, be prepared to wrap up your acceptance over the phone. Most unmatched seniors are placed within a day, many within the first hour.

Beware of programs that stall on making a commitment to you. Remember that this is as difficult a time for program directors as it is for you. Many programs hope to find the best unmatched resident they can, and they may be waiting on someone else. Your waiting on them for a position they want to give to someone else may cost you a spot at a program you would be perfectly happy with. If you are in the Scramble, don't do anything desperate—but at the same time, don't be too picky. Sometimes you have to take what you can get if you really want to be an intern next year. On the other hand, you are not obligated to enter any residency program if you don't want to. If you really had your heart set on a certain city or specialty and it didn't work out, consider taking a year off, bolstering your application, and trying again next year. After all the years of schooling you've put into medicine, one year off will not kill you.

CHAPTER 13

After the Match

THE DAY AFTER

Congratulations! The Match is over, and a new day is beginning. The day after the Match may be a time of celebration, introspection, or planning. You now know where you will be for the next several years and perhaps for much longer. For most students, however, this day will signal the need to start thinking about moving, finding a house or an apartment, and saying one's good-byes.

Thank-you notes to those who helped you are polite and preserve productive relationships.

Although relatively few students think about "thank you's" so soon after the Match is over, now is the appropriate time to personally thank all your advisers and letter writers. Some busy faculty and community physicians may not even be aware that Match Day has passed, but they are likely to be interested in what happened to you. Others may not be able find out where you matched even if they tried to get Match Day results. Therefore, it is your obligation to tell them. At the very least, a thank-you note is in order. Continuing to maintain a positive relationship with your medical school will serve as your foundation throughout your career.

Your new program director might also like to hear from you after the Match, although it may be advisable to wait a day or two for things to settle down in the residency program office. A list of first-year matched residents is usually available shortly after Match Day. Specific scheduling issues, if critical, should be discussed shortly after the Match—for example, scheduling your upcoming wedding. In addition, ask your program what information or credentials it needs to receive from you. Some of the more academic programs have prerequisite reading that must be completed before the program begins. It's also important to ask about your program's Advanced Cardiac Life Support/Advanced Trauma Life Support (ACLS/ATLS) training policy. Some programs expect you to arrive with certification in hand; others will put you through an ACLS course when you start.

WHAT IF I'M NOT HAPPY WITH MY MATCH RESULT?

The good news is that more than 80% of U.S. seniors get one of their first three choices in the Match. Even if you did not match at one of your top choices, you should have few regrets if you followed the two cardinal matching rules outlined in Chapter 12.

Second thoughts about your match are normal. Just remember not to act on them.

Now that success has been achieved, you might feel as though you are in over your head, particularly if you have chosen to enter a highly prestigious (or infamous) program. Rest assured that the vast majority of students complete residency training successfully. Furthermore, if a residency program judged that you were capable and qualified by accepting you in the Match, they are very likely to have been correct. So this should be a time to relax—not to spend another month in an ICU or taking an ECG book to the beach in June. Taking some time off (especially right after the Match) can be a great idea. You will certainly be busy enough once residency starts!

Although it is rarely appropriate to switch to a different program within the same specialty, students may have second thoughts about the program to which they have matched. This might occur because a family member has become ill and the student needs to return home. Alternatively, a student may become convinced that he or she has chosen the wrong specialty and wants to forestall a multiyear mistake. Should you find yourself in one of these situations, you must go see your new program director in person and explain your circumstances. Although you are legally obligated to remain in the program to which you have matched for at least one year, most program directors have students' best interests at heart and are sympathetic to extraordinary circumstances that may arise.

THE RESIDENCY CONTRACT

After the Match, you will receive a residency contract that you must sign and return to your program. The Accreditation Council for Graduate Medical Education (ACGME) recommends that certain terms and conditions be clearly addressed in the contract (see Table 13-1). Before you sign your contract, understand the definitions of all essential terms.

You will also begin to receive a large number of forms from your residency program. As obvious as it may sound, **open** your mail as it is received! Try to stay on top of these forms to help ensure a smooth transition into your internship. You will likely receive a vacation request form and an elective request form. Remember that your vacation weeks will usually fall during your elective or outpatient rotations, so think about when you might want to schedule a lighter month or have to travel (e.g., for weddings or graduation ceremonies). You might also want to organize essential documents into a file. Items such as proof of citizenship (e.g., birth certificate, passport, or Social Security card) as well as ACLS and BCLS (Basic Cardiac Life Support) certificates are useful to have on hand. You are also likely to need a head shot (you can use your ERAS application picture) for your residency program's composite. It is a good idea to print a hard copy of all your application materials (from ERAS and the NRMP site) after the Match, as this information will disappear when the new applicants come along.

LOANS

It is a good idea to get a handle on your student loans now so that you will not have to spend as much time thinking about them during your busy internship year. Most U.S. medical schools' financial aid offices will conduct "exit interviews" in which they will provide information, resources, and strategies for dealing with your loans. Be sure to come to this exit interview prepared—know your loan type and amount, lender, interest rates, and loan features (e.g., grace period, deferment, capitalization). Also, bring a permanent or family home address where your loan paperwork can be sent if you are in the process of moving. The better prepared you are, the easier it will be for you to understand your repayment options and arrange them with your financial aid officer.

It is very important that the demands of the intern year do not result in missing due dates for deferment or forbearance applications or overlooking the end of your grace period for your loans. Mark a date a month in advance on your calendar or PDA to remind yourself of the upcoming deadlines. Forms often take up to three weeks for delivery and processing, so simply meeting a postmark deadline won't always be adequate.

TABLE 13-1.
Essential Residency Contract Terms

Resident's responsibilities
Salary and other stipends
Other benefits
Length of contract and terms of renewal
Policies for sick leave, parental leave, etc.
Grievance and sexual harassment policies

Before starting residency can be a good time to organize your finances.

Moving right along, your next priority is relocating. Nobody enjoys this process, but it doesn't have to be horrible. Some choice pointers follow.

Housing Tips

Housing should be arranged before graduation if at all possible. Your first step should be to explore the pros and cons of renting versus buying, since housing costs vary widely across the United States, and a good deal for one area may not be your best bet in another. Often, the best approach is to talk to members of the current house staff at your program to get their impressions of the local market. As long as you can afford the payments, buying a small home or a condo may make investment sense if you plan to stay in the area for several years. On the other hand, renting will give you the flexibility to look for bigger and better places after you have had a chance to size up the area. For the first year, it's important to focus on finding a short commute and a hassle-free situation, as every hour is precious during internship.

If you are moving with a partner, you might consider making a list of housing options and features and prioritizing the list into "must haves" and "can live without." For example, knowing that you couldn't live without a dishwasher but can compromise with a small yard is important for narrowing your search.

There are many ways to find housing opportunities: You can call up friends who live near the program for housing tips; ask the residency office about housing options; visit a realty or a professional rental service (ask your program or other residents for referrals); go to the local library to look at the classifieds section in local newspapers; or use the Internet to search for available housing in your new city. Listings available through rental and roommate agencies tend to be of higher quality, since the listing fee is self-selecting. Unless it's a huge hassle, plan to visit the city for at least two to four days to find and finalize housing arrangements. If the market is really hot, it is best to come prepared to settle or sign a lease during your visit. During this time, check with a second- or third-year resident to get a local opinion about your choice.

Moving Tips

In anticipation of your move, prepare change-of-address cards and arrange mail forwarding with your local post office. Keep a list of bills you receive during the last few months before you move, and fill out the change-of-address form (or call) when you make your payments. For tracking and insurance purposes, you should catalog your belongings (if you have a lot of material, you might organize it by room) and photograph valuable items. Selling or donating all nonessential belongings will streamline both your move and your life in the long run. In addition, make sure you have adequate packing materials before you start the job (see Table 13-2). Many grocery stores, book stores, or liquor stores will donate large cardboard boxes that are sturdy enough for packing books. Furniture stores are typically more than happy to supply you with boxes or large sheets of leftover plastic and bubble wrap.

TABLE 13-2. Packing Essentials Checklist

☐ Packing boxes

☐ Newspapers

☐ Plastic/bubble wrap

☐ Cord/rope

☐ Packing tape

☐ Scissors

☐ Utility knife

☐ Markers

☐ Labels

You have several options for moving your belongings once you have packed. If you have little or no furniture (or none worth taking), your move will be easy; just pack your unbreakable belongings and call UPS at (800) PICK-UPS for a pickup. UPS does have a limit on the maximum size and weight per box, so call for details. The company automatically insures goods for up to $100 per box and sells insurance for belongings of greater value. Move your valuable or more fragile items personally.

UPS and PODS are alternatives to U-Haul and traditional movers.

If you have furniture worth keeping, you might want to consider moving it yourself. There are a number of self-moving companies with one-way moving vans, including Ryder and U-Haul. If you contact a local branch of such a company rather than the central office, you can often bargain for the truck/van rental. This is the cheaper way to move, but beware of the hassle factor. Another option is PODS (portable on-demand storage), where you pack and unpack but delivery is provided. This service is not provided in all areas, but for a complete listing and more information, visit the Web site www.pods.com. It's also worth considering hiring professional movers to do the job; although it will cost more, you won't be adding the stress of moving to the stress associated with starting your internship. Just be sure to carefully look over any contract you sign for all the terms and conditions (especially about delivery).

Settling Down

By all means take a vacation, but give yourself at least one or two weeks to settle into your new home before your internship starts. You will need this block of time to set up your household, open bank accounts, turn on utilities, and install a telephone line. If you show up two days before a busy internship begins, it may take you the next two months just to unpack. Keep in mind that you and your future co-interns may want time for informal get-togethers before orientation technically starts. Extra time will also give you a chance to explore your new neighborhood and city before internship takes over your life. You won't want to waste time later locating grocery stores, affordable restaurants, 24-hour gas stations, and the like. Try to streamline all nonmedical aspects of your life (e.g., bill paying, shopping) so that what little time off you have during internship ends up being "quality time."

There is no better time to simplify your life.

LICENSING

The Match is over, and you've moved into a nice apartment five minutes from the hospital. Now all you have to do is brace for internship, right?

Well . . . almost. At some point during your residency, you will have to apply for licensure, the USMLE Step 3, and DEA registration. For most new physicians, licensure is most often left until the last months of training, but having your documents in order before residency starts is always a good idea—and keeps your vacation time free from frenzied searches for important credentials. These applications require that you fill out a mountain of paperwork and involve notarized documents, fingerprints, and birth certificates. Thus, the preparation you begin before starting your internship will minimize your stress and vastly enhance your ability to become licensed when you want to be or are required to be.

Resources available on the Internet include www.physicianlicensing.com and www.healthcarelicensing.com. Armed with this information, you will be able to control all three of these critical processes so that you can become licensed in a timely fashion with a minimum number of surprises (e.g., deadlines, exam dates, and required fees).

What Is Licensure?

"Licensure" is the legal term that denotes approval to practice medicine. It is granted by a governing body on the basis of the laws in your jurisdiction. Some states offer several types of licensure—e.g., training, military, inactive, locum tenens, temporary, or permanent. Periods of licensure also vary from state to state; some licenses are valid for only one year, others for two. Similarly, some licenses can be renewed after a set period of time that is based on your birth date, while others are renewable on an annual basis during a particular month of the year. All 50 states require applicants to have successfully passed the USMLE Steps 1, 2 (CK and CS), and 3 exams in order to be eligible for licensure. Since each state has a different fee, the cost of the entire process varies, but plan on putting aside at least $2600 for all three USMLE Steps, and around $1500 for the application process.

You should also be aware that in some states, the medical board can fine residents and programs up to $2500 for failing to obtain licensure as defined by the law. In support of this legislation, some programs have been known to terminate house staff who fail to become licensed by state-mandated deadlines.

In addition, medical boards process thousands of applications each year, usually on a first-come, first-served basis. They will not process files that are out of order for any reason whatsoever. So be courteous when discussing your application with licensing technicians, and allow for plenty of time.

Steps Toward Licensure

The following tips will help further your goal of obtaining licensure in a straightforward and timely manner. Once you have matched, we recommend that you obtain the regulations for licensure in the state where you will be training. Then carefully review those regulations, paying particular attention to when the USMLE Step 3 exam dates and deadlines are, when you are eligible for licensure, and when you are required to be licensed in your jurisdiction. Then start the licensure application process six months before the licensure deadline in your state. Before you Perma-Plaque or frame your medical school diploma, be sure to make ten copies of it on $8^{1}/_{2}$- by 11-inch paper. Send all forms via certified, registered, or express mail, or enclose prepaid postcards to allow for acknowledgment of materials received. When dealing with medical board personnel, be very courteous (they're just like residency application secretaries: cross them and you're history), and be honest about your background.

WHAT'S NEEDED

Table 13-3 summarizes the most common materials requested by state medical boards for licensure. Once you know what is required for licensure in

TABLE 13-3. Items Commonly Requested by State Medical Licensing Boards as Requirements for Medical Licensure

Medical school diploma (either original diploma or an official copy with the registrar's signature and school seal)
Official medical school transcript
Official undergraduate school transcript
Two to three recently taken passport photographs
Two to three letters of recommendation
Letter from residency program director
Official USMLE Steps 1, 2, and 3 score reports
Fingerprints
Completed application with notarized signature
Application fee (usually around $600–$1000)
Letter of good standing from any other state licensing boards from which you were granted licensure

your jurisdiction, you can prepare for the application process by doing some or all of the following, as appropriate:

- Identify the location and cost of photographic services. Be sure to find a photographic service near your place of work, as you may need to make a few visits there during work hours.
- Identify the location and cost of a notary public. If there is no notary public in your facility, try real-estate offices or banks. Be aware, however, that many notary publics have limited hours of availability. Also be sure to complete your application before obtaining notarization, but do not sign the application until you are in the presence of the notary. A valid picture ID will also be required—e.g., a driver's license or a passport.
- Identify the location and cost of fingerprinting services.
- Identify potential personal references, and then contact them to discuss their willingness to serve as references on your behalf.
- Research the addresses and costs of obtaining academic transcripts.
- List all hospitals and addresses where staff privileges have been granted.
- Order a certified copy of your birth certificate.
- If you have changed your name, locate and obtain documentation that will verify that change.

Obstacles to Licensure

Potential obstacles to licensure that both U.S. graduates and international medical graduates (IMGs) may face are as follows:

- **Missing critical deadlines** (e.g., failure to apply for and take the USMLE Step 3 in conjunction with licensing deadlines). Since one of the primary requirements for licensure is successful passage of the USMLE Step 3 examination, you must time Step 3 so that you take it at least three months prior to your licensure deadline. This will allow for the scoring of your exam as well as for the reporting of your scores to the medical board. Another benefit of taking the exam early is that it allows you time to take it again should that prove necessary.

- **Failure to include correct licensure/exam fees along with your application.** Most medical boards will return your application if the fees you enclosed are incorrect. You should also be aware that most application fees are nonrefundable.

- **Failure to provide complete and accurate information on your application.** In reviewing your application, medical boards sometimes uncover discrepancies such as inconsistently reported attendance dates. If this is the case, the board must write you a letter explaining the discrepancy they found and what you must do to rectify it.

- **Incomplete documentation.** As is the case with all bureaucracies, forms are not always completed properly by other institutions. Unfortunately, however, incomplete forms sent to the medical board by your undergraduate school, medical school, or training program will be returned to you to correct. You may then need to call the facility where the error occurred to ensure that the forms are properly handled the second time around.

- **Submitting unrequested documentation to the medical board.** Documents that have not been requested but are enclosed with your application can confuse and frustrate licensing technicians. Moreover, the inclusion of such documents in your application package can raise troubling questions both about your application and about your ability to follow basic instructions.

- **Administrative holds on transcripts.** Transcripts can be held for a variety of reasons, including delinquent student loans, unpaid library fines, and the like.

- **Administrative holds by training programs.** Program directors may deny your request to complete your licensure form on the basis of factors such as incomplete patient chart dictations. (This is rare, but it has been known to occur.)

- **Disregarding requests for additional documentation.** Requests for additional documentation by the medical board are commonplace but should not be ignored, as some states consider a file closed if it has not been fully completed within a certain period of time. You should provide all documentation requested in a timely manner.

- **Failing to report a change of address to the medical board.** Most states will not forward licenses in the mail. Thus, if you have recently moved, be sure to notify your medical board of your new address in writing at the earliest possible time.

- **Failing to keep copies of documents that are submitted to the medical board.** It is always a good idea to keep extra copies of all forms and their addresses. This will help you track lost documents and will also help resolve questions the board might have on a particular document.

- **Exhibiting abusive behavior toward medical board personnel.** Medical board personnel typically have a very large workload. Thus, working cooperatively with them is clearly in your best interests. Remember, board personnel don't make the licensing laws; they're just chartered to uphold them.

- **Starting the application process too late.** If you are not licensed by the deadline set by your state medical board, you may be unable to continue your training program.

The following potential obstacles to licensure apply to IMGs only:

- **Getting forms completed by a foreign medical school.** Documents sent to foreign medical schools often require additional processing time. It can thus be highly advantageous to have someone living near your medical school oversee the process of document completion, mailing, and the like.
- **Failure to complete sufficient hours in required clinical rotations.** IMGs should carefully review licensing requirements for the state from which they are requesting licensure.
- **Inadequate documentation of individual clinical rotations.** Some states have their own individual forms to be used for documenting each rotation. Again, contact your medical board for details.
- **Failure to use medical-board-approved translators for documents written in other languages.** Some state medical boards have a list of translators whom they have deemed acceptable for translating application documents. Contact your medical board for more information.

The USMLE Step 3

To apply for Step 3, you must meet the following requirements before submitting an application:

1. Meet the Step 3 requirements set by the medical licensing authority to which you are applying.
2. Obtain your MD degree (or the equivalent) or DO degree.
3. Receive a passing score on Step 1 and Step 2.
4. If you are an IMG, obtain certification by the Educational Commission for Foreign Medical Graduates (ECFMG) or complete a "fifth pathway" program.

Most states will also require that you have completed or have almost completed one year of postgraduate training in a residency program accredited by the ACGME.

When you send in your application for Step 3, you will not be given the option to select a time period within which you wish to take the exam (as was the case for Steps 1 and 2). Instead, you should allow four to six weeks for the processing of your application. When this is completed, a scheduling permit will be sent to you. You may then schedule a test date. The Step 3 exam is available throughout the year except for two weeks in January. Because Step 3 is a two-day exam that must be taken on consecutive business days, it is important both to schedule your test date as soon as you receive your scheduling permit and to keep your appointment. As with Steps 1 and 2, Step 3 uses computer-based testing. For general information on licensure and Step 3, contact:

Federation of State Medical Boards of the United States, Inc.
P.O. Box 619850
Dallas, TX 75261-9850
Main phone: (817) 868-4000
Main fax: (817) 868-4099
www.fsmb.org

Plan ahead for the USMLE Step 3. Although the cost of taking the exam is $635 (for the year 2006), some states add administrative charges to the overall cost. Moreover, these extra charges can vary from state to state since some state medical boards conduct the Step 3 examination themselves while others rely on the USMLE to do so. In addition, the cost usually increases from year to year (the current cost is set to cap at $660 for 2007). The application for Step 3 also differs somewhat from those for the USMLE Steps 1 and 2—e.g., your signature must be notarized, and additional documents may be required. Faxed documents are unacceptable, but you can use Express Mail, Federal Express, or UPS to deliver your application. Be sure to make copies of all documents, and allow for the six to eight weeks required to score the exam. Listed below are some basic administrative guidelines to follow when preparing to take the USMLE Step 3:

- **Contact the FSMB or call your state medical board for a USMLE Step 3 application, and read it carefully.** Experience has taught that it is critical to verify when you are eligible to take the Step 3 exam, as this may vary from state to state.
- **Start the application process early.** Begin pulling together your supporting documentation as soon as possible.
- **Find out when your state requires you to be licensed and whether that date differs from that of your training program's requirement.** To help you determine when to take Step 3, work backward from your state licensure deadline to determine when you should schedule the exam. Be sure to factor in the six to eight weeks that it will take for scoring and notification of results.
- **Locate a photographic service for required application photos.**
- **Identify a notary public in your facility to obtain required notarizations.**
- **Oh, yeah—don't forget to study.**

For more information, refer to *First Aid for the® USMLE Step 3.*

DON'T FORGET TO WRITE

Congratulations! You've made it to internship. We hope that the advice and information in this book was helpful. Much of what you have read comes from the experiences of students who have gone before you. We hope you'll share the lessons you have learned with those who follow by e-mailing us or sending in the contribution forms in the front of this book. As for internship, nothing can save you from that. But don't worry—in a year, you'll be done. Best of luck!

Reference

Federation of State Medical Boards (FSMB) Web site (www.fsmb.org).

Appendix A

Additional copies of this worksheet are available for download at www. FirstAidfortheBoards.com.

Directions: Fill in blanks below with requested numbers/names/dates. Under **Application Requirements**, list each requirement by name. Once you have assembled the item for that application, check it off.

Program Name	Application Mailing Address	Contact & Phone #	App. Deadline	Application Requirements	Notes
				☐ ☐ ☐ ☐ ☐	
				☐ ☐ ☐ ☐ ☐	
				☐ ☐ ☐ ☐ ☐	
				☐ ☐ ☐ ☐ ☐	
				☐ ☐ ☐ ☐	

Directions: Fill in blanks below with requested numbers/names/dates. Under **Application Requirements**, list each requirement by name. Once you have assembled the item for that application, check it off.

Program Name	Application Mailing Address	Contact & Phone #	App. Deadline	Application Requirements	Notes
				☐ ☐ ☐ ☐ ☐	
				☐ ☐ ☐ ☐ ☐	
				☐ ☐ ☐ ☐ ☐	
				☐ ☐ ☐ ☐ ☐	
				☐ ☐ ☐ ☐ ☐	

Directions: Fill in blanks below with requested numbers/names/dates. Under **Application Requirements**, list each requirement by name. Once you have assembled the item for that application, check it off.

Program Name	Application Mailing Address	Contact & Phone #	App. Deadline	Application Requirements	Notes
				☐ ☐ ☐ ☐ ☐	
				☐ ☐ ☐ ☐ ☐	
				☐ ☐ ☐ ☐ ☐	
				☐ ☐ ☐ ☐ ☐	
				☐ ☐ ☐ ☐ ☐	

Directions: Fill in blanks below with requested numbers/names/dates. Under **Application Requirements**, list each requirement by name. Once you have assembled the item for that application, check it off.

Program Name	Application Mailing Address	Contact & Phone #	App. Deadline	Application Requirements	Notes
				☐ ☐ ☐ ☐ ☐	
				☐ ☐ ☐ ☐ ☐	
				☐ ☐ ☐ ☐ ☐	
				☐ ☐ ☐ ☐ ☐	
				☐ ☐ ☐ ☐ ☐	

Directions: Fill in blanks below with requested numbers/names/dates. Under **Application Requirements**, list each requirement by name. Once you have assembled the item for that application, check it off.

Program Name	Application Mailing Address	Contact & Phone #	App. Deadline	Application Requirements	Notes
				☐ ☐ ☐ ☐ ☐	
				☐ ☐ ☐ ☐ ☐	
				☐ ☐ ☐ ☐ ☐	
				☐ ☐ ☐ ☐ ☐	
				☐ ☐ ☐ ☐	

Appendix B

PROGRAM EVALUATION WORKSHEET (PEW)

Additional copies of this worksheet are available for download at www. FirstAidfortheBoards.com.

Program Name _____

Date of Visit _____

Factor	Comments
Location	
Setting	
Reputation	
Stability of program	
Subspecialty strengths	
Education	
Conferences/rounds	
Faculty teaching	
Postresidency plans of graduates	
Research/teaching opportunities	
Work Environment	
Patient population/load	
Patient responsibilities	
Call frequency/ hours per week	
Ancillary support (e.g., nursing)	
On-call support (e.g., night float, admission caps)	
Health benefits	
Non-health benefits	
Vacation/sick leave/ parenting leave	

Other Factors/Notes

Gut feeling

Advantages	Disadvantages

Preliminary Rank

☐ Top third   ☐ Middle third   ☐ Bottom third   ☐ Do not rank

Interview Log

Name/Address	Notes

Index

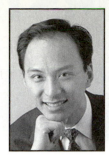
Tao Le, MD, MHS

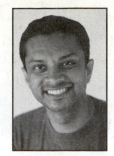
Vikas Bhushan, MD

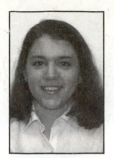
April Troy, MPH

Tao Le, MD, MHS   Tao has been a well-recognized figure in medical education for the past 15 years. As senior editor, he has led the expansion of *First Aid* into a global educational series. In addition, he is editor-in-chief and founder of the *USMLERx* online test bank series as well as a cofounder of the *Underground Clinical Vignettes* series. As a medical student, he was editor-in-chief of the University of California, San Francisco *Synapse*, a university newspaper with a weekly circulation of 9000. Tao earned his medical degree from the University of California, San Francisco and completed his residency training in internal medicine at Yale University and fellowship training at Johns Hopkins University in allergy and immunology. At Yale, he was a regular guest lecturer on the USMLE review courses and an adviser to the Yale University School of Medicine curriculum committee. Tao subsequently went on to co-found Medsn and served as its chief medical officer. He is currently an assistant clinical professor conducting research in asthma education at the University of Louisville.

Vikas Bhushan, MD   Vikas is an author, editor, entrepreneur, and roaming teleradiologist who divides his days between Los Angeles, Maui, and balmy remote locales with abundant bandwidth. In 1992 he conceived and authored the original *First Aid for the USMLE Step 1*, and in 1998 he originated and coauthored the *Underground Clinical Vignettes* series. His entrepreneurial adventures include a successful software company; a medical publishing enterprise (S2S); an e-learning company (Medsn); and, most recently, an ER teleradiology venture (24/7 Radiology). His eclectic interests include medical informatics, independent film, humanism, Urdu poetry, world music, South Asian diasporic culture, and avoiding a day job. He has also coproduced a music documentary on qawwali; coproduced and edited *Shabash 2.0: The Hip Guide to All Things South Asian in North America* (available at www.artwallah.org/shabash); and is now completing a CD/book project on Sufi poetry translated into four languages. Vikas completed a bachelor's degree in biochemistry from the University of California, Berkeley; an MD with thesis from the University of California, San Francisco; and a radiology residency from the University of California, Los Angeles.

April Troy, MPH   April is currently a fourth-year medical student at Johns Hopkins University School of Medicine. She completed her undergraduate education at the University of Scranton. During medical school, she has been very active in the Baltimore community with various community service projects and also serves on the school's Interaction Council, a group which helps students interested in community service at Hopkins. She recently completed a master's degree in public health from Johns Hopkins Bloomberg School of Public Health. She hopes to pursue a career in pediatrics.

ABOUT THE AUTHORS

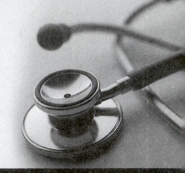